DENTISTRY AND ORAL SCIENCES

SCENARIO BASED MCQ IN DENTISTRY

Dentistry and Oral Sciences

Additional books and e-books in this series can be found on Nova's website under the Series tab.

DENTISTRY AND ORAL SCIENCES

SCENARIO BASED MCQ IN DENTISTRY

MOHAMMAD KHURSHEED ALAM
KIRAN KUMAR GANJI
BADER K. ALZAREA
SANTOSH R. PATIL
AND
MOHAMMED G. SGHAIREEN
EDITORS

nova
Medicine & Health
New York

Library of Congress Cataloging-in-Publication Data

ISBN: 978-1-53617-298-0

Published by Nova Science Publishers, Inc. † New York

CONTENTS

PREFACE

Dentistry has constantly evolved over the years to keep abreast of the latest trends, techniques, and diagnostic procedures. Dental Schools have undergone a number of changes in an effort to arrive upon the ideal format for testing clinical knowledge in examinations. Multiple-choice questions (MCQs) have been the most common modality by which dental students were examined. Although MCQs enable the testing of a broad range of topics, as well as being cost effective, they have largely been abandoned in favour of scenario-based questions (SBQs).

Traditional MCQs often abstract and measure only whether people recall facts in their short-term memory. Converting these questions to scenario-based questions can increase the level of difficulty, measure higher level thought and providing relevant context. The authors of *Scenario Based MCQ in Dentistry* have endeavoured to keep these facts in mind and provide a significant number of high-quality SBQs that comprehensively examine the dental curriculum. Most of the questions are scenario based. Each question not only provides an opportunity to apply clinical knowledge and correctly identify the single best answer to a question, but also to learn why the other answers are wrong, greatly increasing the clinical acumen and learning opportunity of the reader.

Selection tests and competitive exams are hurdles that a candidate seeks to clear with ease. It all depends on meticulous preparation and the quality of resource materials available to the student. Considering the quantity of subject matter that needs to be covered, it becomes a herculean task unless the candidate chooses the right training tool. Reference texts are often too advanced and undergraduate texts are insufficiently updated or lacking in depth and detail. In this context, a lack of good revision aids can be frustrating.

This book has been compiled with the selection tests in mind as a tool for rapid revision and analytical learning. It is useful for doctors, dental students, graduates, dental nurses, technicians, as well as specialists seeking professional excellence, or for those studying for the various licensing exams conducted by SCFHS, Saudi Board, HAAD, OMSB, SCHQ, DHCC, DHA, and MOH. This book aims to provide dental students with a useful source for exam preparation, as well as for supplementing the readers' knowledge so that they feel fully prepared for the various postgraduate entrance examinations.

In: Scenario Based MCQ in Dentistry ISBN: 978-1-53617-298-0
Editors: M. Khursheed Alam et al.

Chapter 1

SCENARIO BASED MCQS IN ORAL MEDICINE

Rakhi Issrani and Kumar Chandan Srivastava
Oral Medicine, Preventive Dentistry Department,
College of Dentistry, Jouf University, Aljouf, Saudi Arabia

Oral Medicine is a specialty that deals with study of diagnosis and medical management of diseases of oral structures and systemic diseases manifested in the jaw. Therefore, an understanding of the oro-facial diseases is essential to the effective delivery of comprehensive oral care. Keeping this in mind, this question bank is prepared to help the students of undergraduate studies in Dentistry with relevant information as a foundation on which to build such an understanding of the oro-facial diseases for the effective delivery of comprehensive oral care.

The authors have dedicatedly prepared this section of the book, focusing attention on evaluation of various oro-facial abnormalities. This book is designed for those students who have achieved a satisfactory level of competency in diagnostic skills during their introductory clinical years of the dental training programme. The questions include case scenarios that are well structured and designed to adequately meet the curriculum requirements of Oral Medicine at the undergraduate level. The authors have maintained simplicity and readability that would help any beginner and expert alike relish reading and understanding.

We hope this question bank will be a valuable companion and a good guide for undergraduate students of Dentistry along with a useful addition to dental literature.

1. A 43-year-old man comes to the dental clinic with the complaint of difficulty in opening his mouth. Previous dental history reveals burning sensation when eating spicy foods and ulcerations of the oral mucosa. Palpation of buccal mucosa reveals a firm fibrous texture. What is the most likely diagnosis? What do you think the cause of the condition could be?
    A. Leukoplakia; smokeless tobacco pouching
    B. Oral submucous fibrosis; Betel Quid & Arecanut use
    C. Oral submucous fibrosis; Cigarette Smoking
    D. Smokeless tobacco pouch keratosis; smokeless tobacco snuff

2. A patient present with swelling in neck near the angle of mandible on right side which disappear on applying pressure to it. Intraorally a dome-shaped, bluish swelling was present in floor of mouth on right side. Most likely diagnosis of the lesion is
    A. Mucocele
    B. Dermoid cyst
    C. Ranula
    D. Branchial cyst

3. Examination of a child shows enlargement of left side of tongue with small, elevated greyish-pink nodules, some of which are fluid-filled with rest of oral cavity being normal. Most likely diagnosis of the lesion is
    A. Neurofibromatosis
    B. Lymphangioma

C. Granular cell myoblastoma
D. Cystic fibrosis

4. A patient present with small yellow spots, present bilaterally on buccal mucosa opposite to posterior teeth without any other associated complaint. Most probable diagnosis of the condition is
    A. Koplik's spot
    B. Fordyce's granules
    C. Melanotic macule
    D. White sponge nevus

5. A patient present with a bilateral grayish white lesion on buccal mucosa which disappear when stretched. The most likely diagnosis is
    A. Lichen planus
    B. Leukoplakia
    C. Leukoedema
    D. White sponge nevus

6. A 34-year-old female patient came to your clinic with the chief complaint of swelling on the lateral surface of the tongue. The patient gave a history of trauma at the same site 10 years back with no history of associated pain or bleeding from the site. On intraoral examination, there was a growth measuring about 1.5cm × 1.5cm, which was red in color with a bluish hue present at the left lateral surface of the tongue. The growth was soft to palpate, and it showed blanching on application of pressure. What is your provisional diagnosis?
    A. Hemangioma
    B. Lymphangioma
    C. Lipoma
    D. Fibroma

7. A 35-year-old female patient came to your clinic with the chief complaint of dry lips and mouth, bilateral submandibular edema and ocular dryness. What is the probable diagnosis?
   A. Peutz-Jeghers syndrome
   B. Sjogren's syndrome
   C. Grinspan syndrome
   D. McCune-Albright syndrome

8. On palpation, the lymph nodes were found to be rubbery in consistency. What is your probable diagnosis?
   A. Lipoma
   B. Mucocele
   C. Caseating tuberculosis
   D. Lymphomas

9. Twitching of facial muscles following tapping over the facial nerve in front of the ear is suggestive of
   A. Latent tetany in hypoparathyroidism
   B. Latent tetany in hyperparathyroidism
   C. Latent tetany in hypothyroidism
   D. Latent tetany in hyperthyroidism

10. A 24-year-old female has flaccid bullae in the skin and oral erosions. Histopathology shows intra-epidermal acantholytic blisters. The most likely diagnosis is
    A. Pemphigoid
    B. Pemphigus vulgaris
    C. Erythema multiforme
    D. Dermatitis herpatiformis

11. A 45-year-old male has multiple grouped vesicular lesions present on the T10 segment dermatome associated with pain. The most likely diagnosis is
    - **A. Herpes zoster**
    - B. Dermatitis herpetiformis
    - C. Herpes simplex
    - D. Coxsackie infection

12. A 4-year-old child presents with fever, gingival bleeding and extensive oral ulceration in his mouth. His medical history is unremarkable. What would be your most likely diagnosis?
    - A. Candidal infection
    - **B. Herpes simplex infection**
    - C. Recurrent aphthous ulceration
    - D. Herpes zoster infection

13. A 60-year-old patient presented with several bullous lesions for the last 3 days. Each bullous lesion was surrounded by an erythematous halo. There were multiple target lesions. Patient also had oral erosions. The most likely diagnosis is
    - A. Chicken pox
    - B. Herpes simplex
    - C. Herpes zoster
    - **D. Erythema multiforme**

14. A 6-year-old child comes to your clinic with the history of low grade fever, anorexia, diarrhea, vomiting, lymphadenopathy, and pharyngitis. On examination you notice vesicular lesions present bilaterally on the extensor surface of the skin of hands, fingers, feet, toes, tongue, check mucosa, tonsils and pharynx. What is your clinical diagnosis?
    - A. Herpes zoster
    - **B. Hand, foot and mouth disease**
    - C. Herpes simplex type I
    - D. Histoplasmosis

15. The gastric mucosa has the important ability to prevent movement of gastricacid from the stomach lumen into the gastric wall. Some diseases and drug regimen have been implicated as causes of increased gastric mucosal permeability to hydrogen ion. Drugs which may increase gastric wall permeability include
    A. Erythromycin
    B. Epinephrine
    C. Nitrofurantoin
    D. Aspirin

16. An 8-year-old child presented with brownish discolored and deformed anterior teeth. History of having received an antibiotic about 4 years earlier was obtained. Which antibiotic could be responsible for the condition?
    A. Chloramphenicol
    B. Tetracycline
    C. Erythromycin
    D. Penicillin

17. The persistent suppression of bacterial growth that may occur following limited exposure to some antimicrobial drugs is called
    A. Time-dependent killing
    B. Post-antibiotic effect
    C. Clinical synergy
    D. Concentration-dependent killing

18. A patient on antibiotic therapy for scarlet fever develops white plaques on his oral mucosa which when scraped with tongue blade leaves a painful bleeding surface. The most probable diagnosis is
    A. Blastomycosis
    B. Candidiasis
    C. Herpes simplex infection
    D. Syphilis

19. A patient presented with asymptomatic, smooth, circumscribed red area in midline anterior to circumvallate papillae on the dorsum of tongue with microscopic evidence of epithelial hyperplasia. The most probable diagnosis of the condition is
    A. Geographic tongue
    B. Hairy tongue
    C. Median rhomboid glossitis
    D. Lingual thyroid

20. A middle-aged patient complains of periodic burning of her buccal mucosa. Oral examination shows slightly raised, linear, grayish-white plaque present bilaterally on buccal mucosa. Biopsy of the lesion shows acanthosis, surface keratosis with vacuolation of cells of basal cell layer with cellular inflammatory infiltrate localized to sub-epithelial connective tissue. Most likely diagnosis is
    A. Lichen planus
    B. Leokoedema
    C. Luekoplakia
    D. Pemphigoid

21. A patient present with an asymptomatic white corrugated patch present bilaterally on his buccal mucosa. He also reports the occurrence of same kind of lesion in his mother and younger brother. Most likely diagnosis is
    A. Pemphigus
    B. Leukoedema
    C. Candidiasis
    D. White sponge nevus

22. A patient present with erythematosus scaly lesions on extensor aspect of elbows and knee. The clinical diagnosis is achieved by
    A. Auspitz sign
    B. KOH smear
    C. Tzanck smear
    D. Skin biopsy

23. A patient reported with an asymptomatic white patch on buccal mucosa which cannot be rubbed off. The patch was present for the last 3 months. Patient is a heavy cigarette smoker. Most probable diagnosis of the lesion is
    A. Leukoplakia
    B. Candidiasis
    C. Erythroplakia
    D. White sponge nevus

24. A 27-year-old female reported to the dental clinic with a complaint of recurring and subsiding burning sensation in the mouth and sensitivity to hot and spicy food for the last 8 months. She also complains of red areas on the tongue concomitant to the burning sensation and disappearance of the red areas when burning subsides. Oral examination reveals multiple demarcated zones of erythema on the tongue. These zones are surrounded by slightly elevated serpentine, white borders. What do you think would be the most appropriate diagnosis?
    A. Erythematosus candidiasis
    B. Erythematosus oral lichen planus
    C. Erythroplakia
    D. Geographic tongue

25. A 30-year-old patient reported to dental clinic with the chief complaint of lesion on her tongue. She had similar lesions at the same site previously and they healed in a couple of weeks. Which of the following lesions should head your list of differential diagnosis?
    A. Recurrent aphthous ulcer
    B. Recurrent herpes simplex infection
    C. Ectopic geographic tongue
    D. Oral lichen planus

26. A 55-year-old female presents with severe, electrical and shocking pain in her right cheek triggered by light touch. Clinical examination

does not reveal any local cause. Which drug is most likely to be effective for her?

A. Baclofen
B. Ergotamine
C. Carbamazepine
D. Paracetamol

27. A 45-year-old female presents with a 6 months' history of recurrent mealtime swelling and pain in the floor of her mouth. Clinical examination does not reveal any dental abnormality. What is the most likely cause of her symptoms?

A. Lymphadenitis
B. Sialolithiasis
C. Sialorrhea
D. Xerostomia

28. A 65-year-old male presents to you for dental treatment for a rapidly growing ulcerated and indurated lesion. He is a chronic chain smoker (20 cigarettes per day). On examination, a hard, fixed, non-tender submandibular lymph node is palpable. Which lesion would you suspect to run further investigations?

A. Oral squamous cell carcinoma
B. Spread of dental infection (abscess) to larynx
C. Severe tonsillitis
D. Lymphadenopathy of jugulo-omohyoid region

29. A 40-year-old male presents to you with paroxysmal, sharp, lancinating pain affecting one side of the throat and base of the tongue that is precipitated by swallowing, chewing and coughing. The most probable diagnosis in this case is

A. Trigeminal neuralgia
B. Glossopharyngeal neuralgia
C. Post herpetic neuralgia
D. Frey's syndrome

30. "You seem to be making progress, don't you agree?" is an example of which method of collecting patient data?
    A. Asking leading questions
    B. Asking hypothetical questions
    C. Asking closed-ended questions
    D. Asking open-ended questions

31. A 2cm discrete, white lesion of the buccal mucosa has not resolved after elimination of all local irritations. The most appropriate management would be to
    A. Cauterize it
    B. Apply toluidine blue staining
    C. Perform an incisional biopsy
    D. Re-examine at 6-month interval

32. A female patient complains of pain in right ear radiating towards the angle of mandible. Clicking sounds were present in right temporomandibular joint. Results of palpation and radiographic examination are negative. The most probable diagnosis is
    A. Osteoarthritis
    B. Rheumatoid arthritis
    C. Myofacial pain dysfunction syndrome
    D. Traumatic arthritis

33. You suspect that your patient has an enlarged submandibular salivary gland. You expect the enlarged gland
    A. to be palpable intraorally
    B. to be palpable extraorally
    C. to be palpable both intra- and extraorally
    D. only to be detectable by radiographic examination

34. Which muscle is the most active during a right lateral excursion of the mandible?
    A. Left lateral pterygoid muscle
    B. Right lateral pterygoid muscle

C. Left medial pterygoid muscle
D. Right medial pterygoid muscle

35. A 32-year-old patient came to the dental clinic. Dentist asks her about the medical and dental history for leading to the examination and diagnosis for management of her condition. Which one the following is not a meaning of the history taking?
    A. The initial part of the discussing between the dentist and patient
    B. The dentist asks the mother for the patient's first visit to a hospital
    C. The dentist should have an idea of the patient's concerns
    D. The dentist should use methodical questioning to elucidate further details

36. A 40-year-old male patient reported to your dental clinic with the chief complaint of swollen lips. All of the following are the causes of large lip *except*
    A. Acromegaly
    B. Chelitis glandularis
    C. Cretinism
    D. Peutz-Jeghers syndrome

37. A 25-year-old male patient visited your clinic with a chief complaint of an ulcer on tip of the tongue. On examination, the ulcer was found to be soft, with undermined edges and serosanguineous discharge was observed. What is the most probable diagnosis?
    A. Syphilitic ulcer
    B. Rodent ulcer
    C. Tubercular ulcer
    D. Malignant ulcer

38. A 39-year-old patient reported to your clinic with the chief complaint of gingival hyperplasia. On asking the medical history, he informed you that he is taking medicine for some medical ailment. All of the following drugs are responsible for gingival hyperplasia *except*
    A. Dilantin
    B. Nifedipine
    C. Cyclosporin
    D. Adrenaline

39. A 60-year-old male presents with unilateral facial paralysis, cutaneous lesions of external meatus hearing defects, and vertigo. What would be your most likely diagnosis?
    A. Bell's palsy
    B. Melkerson Rosenthal syndrome
    C. Ramsay Hunt syndrome
    D. Trigeminal neuralgia

40. A 9-year-old child has multiple itchy erythematous wheals all over the body since 2 days. There is no respiratory difficulty. Which is the best treatment?
    A. Systemic corticosteroids
    B. Anthelminthic
    C. Adrenaline
    D. Antihistamines

41. A 62-year-old patient reported to your clinic with complaint of burning sensation of tongue. This condition is called:
    A. Glossopyrosis
    B. Glossodynia
    C. Glossitis
    D. Glossolgia

42. A 12-year-old child with congenital heart disease came for extraction of his mandibular first molar. The antibiotic of choice for prevention of infective endocarditis is:
    A. Ampicillin 30mg/kg orally 1 hour before procedure
    B. Amoxicillin 50mg/kg orally 1 hour before procedure
    C. Cephalexin 50mg/kg orally 1 hour before procedure
    D. Clindamycin 20mg/kg orally 1 hour before procedure

43. A 36-year-old male patient came to the dental clinic with the chief complaint of erosions at the corner of the lips. The dental history was found to be normal. What is the most likely diagnosis?
    A. Stomatitis
    B. Glossitis migran
    C. Sialadenitis
    D. Cheilitis

44. Patient had anaphylactic shock due to penicillin injection, what is the most important in the emergency treatment to do?
    A. 0.5 mg epinephrine of 1/10000 intravenous
    B. 200mg hydrocortisone intravenous
    C. Adrenaline of 1/1000 intramuscular
    D. 12.5 mg antihistaminic orally

45. Patient comes to your clinic complaining that the denture has become tight. On intraoral examination, everything appeared to be normal, but when the patient stands, you notice that his legs curved. What is your diagnosis?
    A. Cherubism
    B. Paget's disease
    C. Osteosarcoma
    D. Fibrous dysplasia

46. A 25-year-old patient presented to your clinic with an infection and swelling of lymph gland tissue located on both sides of the back of the throat. It is usually caused by virus or, less commonly, a bacterium. The most likely diagnosis is:
    A. Tonsillitis
    B. Gingivitis
    C. Pharyngitis
    D. Glossitis

47. A 58-year-old woman complains of taste dysfunction. Physical examination reveals a loss of taste on the anterior 2/3^{rds} of her tongue which is due to loss of function of:
    A. Chorda tympani nerve
    B. Glossopharyngeal nerve
    C. Vagus nerve
    D. Hypoglossal nerve

48. Patient came to your clinic with the complaint of gingival bleeding even on slight pressure. On clinical examination you found pin point purple dots on palate. Laboratory findings showed decrease in platelets count. This lesion is known as:
    A. Nodule
    B. Tumor
    C. Pustule
    D. Purpura

49. A 60-year-old patient who is a denture wearer comes to your clinic for the routine checkup. On examination, you observe glossitis and angular cheilitis. It could be due to:
    A. Vitamin B deficiency
    B. Scleroderma
    C. Xerostomia
    D. Ptyalism

50. Patient came to your clinic with a lesion confined to the middle of the hard palate. On clinical examination, the lesion was found to be fluctuant and tender. Radiographically, a radiolucent area between the two central incisors was seen. The diagnosis will be:
    - A. Globullomaxillary cyst
    - B. Bohn's nodule
    - C. Epstein pearls
    - **D. Incisive canal cyst**

51. A 58-year-old male presents with hemorrhagic crusting of his lips following a course of antibiotic therapy. He does not have any systemic manifestations. What would be your most likely diagnosis?
    - **A. Erythema Multiforme**
    - B. Anaphylaxis
    - C. Behcet's syndrome
    - D. Lichen Planus

52. Drugs which need certain adjustment and special management before and during dental procedures are:
    - **A. Steroids**
    - B. Anticholinergics
    - C. NSAIDs
    - D. Antihypertensives

53. When a person consents to be an organ donor upon his/her death, what is the most likely procedure that will be performed with the donated organs?
    - A. Xenograft
    - **B. Allograft**
    - C. Isograft
    - D. Autograft

54. The following represents the best pharmacologic therapy for Burning Mouth Syndrome:
    A. Antidepressant agents
    B. Corticosteroids
    C. Anxiolytic agents
    D. There is no therapy of proven general efficacy

55. A 12-year-old male patient presents with a deficiency at the malar bone, open bite and normal mental abilities. What is your most likely diagnosis?
    A. Eagle syndrome
    B. Cleidocranial dysplasia
    C. Treacher-Collins syndrome
    D. Albright's syndrome

56. Trigeminal neuralgia is treated by carbamazepine, the maximum dose per day divided in doses is:
    A. 200mg
    B. 50mg
    C. 1000mg
    D. 1200mg

57. A 32-year-old male patient visited your clinic with a chief complaint of an ulcer on tip of the tongue that was painless. On examination, the ulcer was found to be firm, with sharp edges and wash leather slough was observed on floor of ulcer. What is the most probable diagnosis?
    A. Syphilitic ulcer
    B. Rodent ulcer
    C. Tubercular ulcer
    D. Malignant ulcer

58. A child has ingested an unknown substance and has evidence of respiratory depression. This symptom is usually found with poisoning due to:
    A. Amphetamines

B. Atropine
C. Mushrooms
D. Opioids

59. Where would you document measurable information using SOAP charting?
    A. Objective data
    B. Subjective data
    C. Analysis
    D. Treatment plan

60. A rectal suppository is used to treat a fever. This would represent what type of drug delivery?
    A. Parenteral and local
    B. Parenteral and systemic
    C. Enteral and systemic
    D. Enteral and local

61. Which of the following symptoms is not a recognized feature of classical trigeminal neuralgia?
    A. Light touch provokes the pain
    B. The pain occurs in conjunction with facial flushing
    C. Pain occurs across two divisions of the trigeminal nerve
    D. Severe, shooting pain lasting around 30 seconds

62. A 6-year-old girl is referred to you by a dermatologist for dental treatment. On oral examination, you find hypoplastic teeth, scarring caused by trauma from suckling, eating and tooth brushing resulting into immobility of tongue and lips, cracks at corners of mouth & limited mouth opening. What is the most probable diagnosis is this case?
    A. Mucous membrane pemphigoid
    B. Pemphigus vulgaris
    C. Epidermolysis bullosa
    D. Erosive lichen planus

63. A 44-year-old female presents to you with painless, indurated, dark red swelling in her mouth with glazed surface. These were diagnosed as chancres and Treponema pallidum was isolated from these chancres. The first and second drug of choice for this patient is:
    A. Acyclovir and Fluconazole
    B. Fluconazole and tetracycline
    C. Penicillin and tetracycline or erythromycin
    D. Penicillin only

64. You notice that your patient's submandibular lymph nodes are enlarged. You would look for potential infection sites in the:
    A. Hard palate
    B. Hard palate and upper lip
    C. Hard palate, upper lip and upper central incisor
    D. Hard palate, upper lip, upper central incisor and lower first molar

65. Mid-face hypoplasia, hyperpigmentation, elevated body temperature, protuberant lips, and anodontia are the features of:
    A. Hereditary ectodermal dysplasia
    B. Peutz-Jegher's syndrome
    C. Gardner's syndrome
    D. Sjogren's syndrome

66. The optimum sequence of treatment plan is:
    A. Pretreatment phase, treatment of acute problems, control of active diseases, restoration of esthetics and function, reevaluation of the treatment, recall.
    B. Pretreatment phase, treatment of acute problems, control of active diseases, restoration of esthetics and function, recall, reevaluation of the treatment.
    C. Pretreatment phase, control of active diseases, treatment of acute problems, restoration of esthetics and function, reevaluation of the treatment, recall.

D. Pretreatment phase, treatment of acute problems, control of active diseases, reevaluation of the treatment, restoration of esthetics and function, recall.

67. Atropine:
    A. Dries secretion such saliva
    B. Depresses the pulse rate
    C. Cause central nervous system depression
    D. Cause sleep deprivement

68. Which type of antimicrobial drug combination is most likely to exhibit antagonism?
    A. Bactericidal + bactericidal
    B. Bactericidal + bacteriostatic for a highly sensitive organism
    C. Bactericidal + bacteriostatic for a marginally sensitive organism
    D. Bacteriostatic + bacteriostatic

69. A 10-year-old female presents to you with a rash over her eyelids after using a new cosmetic brand. What is the best test to confirm the cause of the rash?
    A. Punch biopsy
    B. Patch test
    C. Prick skin test
    D. Indirect immunofluorescent antibody test

70. Syphilitic keratosis began with the atrophy of:
    A. Filiform and foliate papillae
    B. Filiform and fungiform papillae
    C. Filiform and circumvallate papillae
    D. Foliate and circumvallate papillae

71. Koebner phenomenon is seen in:
    A. Leukoplakia
    B. Oral Submucous fibrosis
    C. Lichen Planus
    D. Stomatitis nicotina

72. Paterson Kelly syndrome is characterized by the following:
    A. Dysphagia, angular cheilitis and candidiasis
    B. Dysplasia, angular cheilitis and candidiasis
    C. Dysplasia, angular cheilitis and syphilis
    D. Dysphagia, angular cheilitis and syphilis

73. Super-infections are more common with:
    A. Use of narrow spectrum antibiotics
    B. Short courses of antibiotics
    C. Use of antibiotics that are completely absorbed from the small intestine
    D. Use of antibiotic combinations covering both gram positive and gram negative bacteria

74. Acetaminophen has been used as a safe and effective analgesic/antipyreticagent for over 80 years. Since it may be purchased without a prescription, it is readily available and as such the recommended dose may be exceeded. The primary toxicity leading to death from an acetaminophen overdose is:
    A. Papillary necrosis and chronic interstitial nephritis
    B. Pancytopenia
    C. Hepatocellular necrosis
    D. Hemolytic anemia

75. The most frequent cause of xerostomia is:
    A. Aplasia or atresia
    B. Sjogren's syndrome
    C. Drugs
    D. Therapeutic irradiation

76. A patient present with soreness and bleeding of gingivae, necrosis of the gingival papillae and marked halitosis. The drug of choice in this case would be:
    A. Metronidazole 200mg TDS with chlorhexidine mouthwash
    B. Penicillin 500mg T.D.S with amphotericin mouthwash
    C. Chlorhexidine mouthwash with lignocaine gel
    D. Systemic steroids and anti-fungals

77. All of the following are vital signs *except*
    A. Blood pressure
    B. Body temperature
    C. Pulse rate and respiration
    D. Pupil size

78. Percussion of a tooth is used to evaluate: 1. Ankylosis. 2. Pain. 3. Mobility. 4. Vitality.
    A. (1) (2) (3)
    B. (1) and (3)
    C. (2) and (4)
    D. (4) only

79. The following is an example of a true cyst:
    A. Stafne's bone cyst
    B. Traumatic bone cyst
    C. Residual cyst
    D. Aneurysmal bone cyst

80. Burning Mouth Syndrome is a chronic disorder typically characterized by each of the following *except*
    A. Mucosal lesion
    B. Burning pain in multiple oral sites
    C. Pain similar in intensity to toothache pain
    D. Persistent altered taste perception

81. If a patient has symptoms that may indicate more than one condition, what must a doctor do first?
    - **A. Make a differential diagnosis**
    - B. Confirm the patient's overall state of health
    - C. Provide baseline values for vital signs
    - D. Do treatment planning

82. Which of the following drug causes pigmentation of skin?
    - **A. Minocycline**
    - B. Penicillin
    - C. Furosemide
    - D. Amefostine

83. A 46-year-old male patient reported with the chief complaint of pain in his lower left back tooth region of 1-week duration. His medical and dental history was noncontributory. On clinical examination, extraorally and intraorally, no obvious changes were seen in the region of pain. His pantomogram revealed root stumps in relation to maxillary second premolar and a well-defined ovoid radiolucency with sclerotic margin below the inferior alveolar canal and above the lower border of the mandible below the apices of lower second and third molar on the left side was found. Based on the clinical and radiological features, what is your most likely diagnosis?
    - **A. Stafne's cyst**
    - B. Radicular cyst
    - C. Dentigerous cyst
    - D. Residual cyst

84. Behcet's syndrome is characterized by-
    - **A. Oral aphthous ulceration, eye lesions, genital lesions and a positive pathergy test**
    - B. Oral aphthous ulceration, eye lesions, and a positive pathergy test
    - C. Unilateral facial palsy with swelling of the face and lips
    - D. Triad of miosis, ptosis and anhidrosis

85. Healthcare workers may develop what type of herpes lesion if they touch patients or patients' secretions without hand protection?
    A. Cold sores
    B. Herpetic keratitis
    C. A "cigarette burn" pattern of infection
    D. A herpetic whitlow

86. In transillumination test,
    A. A healthy sinus will appear opaque, diseased sinus transmits the light.
    B. A healthy sinus transmits the light, diseased sinus will appear opaque.
    C. A healthy sinus transmits the light completely; diseased sinus will transmits less light.
    D. A healthy sinus transmits will transmits less light, diseased sinus transmits the light completely.

87. What sets the stage for the reactions that occur upon repeated exposure to the same allergen in a type I hypersensitivity reaction?
    A. The release of the allergenic particles into the tissue fluids and lymphatics
    B. Recognition of the allergen by B and T cells
    C. Secretion of IgE by plasma cells
    D. Binding of IgE to mast cells and basophils

88. What is the portal of entry for varicella-zoster virus?
    A. Respiratory epithelium
    B. Mouth
    C. Conjunctiva
    D. Through a break in the skin

89. Inspection by diascopic examination, the following fades under pressure on the glass slide:
    A. Angiomas
    B. Petechiae
    C. Ecchymosis
    D. Macule

90. A 58-year-old female presents with recurrent oral and corneal ulceration. Her biopsy specimen reveals sub-epithelial bullae. What is your most likely diagnosis?
    A. Candidiasis
    B. Squamous cell carcinoma
    C. Mucous membrane pemphigoid
    D. Pemphigus vulgaris

91. Gingival tumor with two contra-lateral mobile lymphnodes in cheek comes under which staging?
    A. T3N2M0
    B. T2N2M0
    C. T4N2M0
    D. T3N3M0

92. Regional lymph node enlargement is present in:
    A. Acute pericoronitis
    B. Lichen planus
    C. Pemphigus vulgaris
    D. Chronic ulcerative stomatitis

93. A 40-year-old female presents with clicking in her right temporomandibular joint (TMJ) for the last six months. She does not have any pain or limitation of her mouth opening. Clinical examination does not reveal odontogenic cause. What does this condition most likely represent?
    A. TMJ ankylosis
    B. Fracture of the mandibular condyle

C. Internal derangement of TMJ
D. Myofascial pain

94. A painful crater-like 1.5 cm ulcer develops within one week on the hard palate mucosa of a 40-yearold female. The most likely diagnosis is:
    A. Actinomycosis
    B. Squamous cell carcinoma
    C. Pleomorphic adenoma
    D. Necrotizing sialometaplasia

95. Waldeyer's ring comprises of:
    A. 1 pharyngeal tonsil, 2 tubal tonsils, 2 palatine tonsils & 1 lingual tonsil
    B. 2 pharyngeal tonsil, 1 tubal tonsils, 1 palatine tonsils & 2 lingual tonsil
    C. 1 pharyngeal tonsil, 2 tubal tonsils, 1 palatine tonsils & 2 lingual tonsil
    D. 1 pharyngeal tonsil, 1 tubal tonsils, 2 palatine tonsils &2 lingual tonsil

96. AIDS is:
    A. Endemic
    B. Epidemic
    C. Pandemic
    D. Sporadic

97. In the clinical evaluation, the most significant finding of the parotid mass may be accompanying:
    A. Rapid progressive painless enlargement
    B. Nodular consistency
    C. Supramental and preauricular lymphadenopathy
    D. Facial paralysis

98. A 60-year-old patient reported to your clinic with an enlargement of left parotid gland that was present since 6 months. On examination, this enlargement was found to be non-inflammatory and non-neoplastic. The term to describe this type of salivary enlargement is:
    - A. Sialadenitis
    - B. Ptyalism
    - **C. Sialosis**
    - D. Sialolith

99. The major concentrations of proprioceptive receptors providing information about position of the TMJ are located in:
    - A. The capsule and ligaments of the TMJ and the medial pterygoid muscle
    - **B. The capsule and ligaments of the TMJ and the lateral pterygoid muscle**
    - C. The articular disc of the TMJ and the medial pterygoid muscle
    - D. The articular disc of the TMJ and the lateral pterygoid muscle

100. A 4-year-old child has a fever of 102° F; and following upper respiratory tract infection, discrete vesicles and ulcers on the soft plate and pharynx are noted. The most probable diagnosis is:
    - A. Scarlet fever
    - **B. Herpangina**
    - C. Herpes zoster
    - D. Herpetic gingivostomatitis

101. A patient after dental extraction showed an immediate reduction in bleeding, but continued to bleed in small amount for the whole day. Which of the investigation will be most appropriate?
    - A. INR
    - **B. Bleeding Time**
    - C. Clotting Time
    - D. Platelet count

102. In which of the following given patient's clinical scenario who will be undergoing a dental extraction, the assessment of coagulation status is not considered as a primary concern in investigations?
    A. Recent history of Viral Hepatitis
    B. History of Stroke followed by regular medication of Antithrombotic drugs
    C. Epileptic patient on a long term carbamazepine therapy
    D. Bronchial asthma

103. On questioning, patient gives a chronic history of wheeze with the exposure of dust and gets relived only with inhalation of drug. Which of the following considerations will be relevant during pre, intra or post-operative phase of dental treatment?
    A. Avoid Non-steroidal anti-inflammatory drugs
    B. Prolonged Bleeding
    C. Antibiotic Prophylaxis
    D. Gingival Enlargement

104. Patient will be considered infective as well as can transmit hepatitis, in case his/her hematology report reflects?
    A. Only Anti HBs
    B. HBsAg with Anti HBs
    C. Anti HBc & Anti HBs
    D. HBsAg without IgM Anti HBc

105. Which of the following statements will be correct for a hypertensive patient receiving LA with adrenalin?
    A. It is an absolute contraindication
    B. Adrenalin injected with LA is less harmful than its endogenous production
    C. It causes peripheral pooling of blood leading to increased risk of hypertension

D. Since adrenalin will increase heart rate by activating parasympathetic system; it will further increase the risk of hypertension

106. A clinician decides to find the number of cases with enamel erosion visiting a dental clinic. The most suitable method of examination with type of dental record to adopted, will be?
    A. Emergency examination with unstructured case record
    B. Screening examination with unstructured case record
    C. Screening examination with structured case record
    D. Emergency examination with structured case record

107. A herpes virus associated red lesion, mostly seen in the hard or soft palate, which is a strongly associated lesion in HIV infection and may be seen with other opportunistic infections as well, is provisionally diagnosed as
    A. Kaposi sarcoma
    B. Atrophic Candidiasis
    C. Hairy Leukoplakia
    D. Gingivostomatitis

108. Which of the following statements is incorrect about corticosteroid?
    A. They are superior Anti-Inflammatory in comparison to NSAID's
    B. Slow and gradual tapering of dosage is required for patient who in on steroid therapy of 10mg/day for the past 1 week
    C. Orabase should be present in all topical preparation of corticosteroid
    D. Clobetasol 17-Propionate is a high potency corticosteroid

109. A congenital, bilateral, keratotic white lesion seen on buccal mucosa will be provisionally diagnosed as
    A. Lichen Planus
    B. White Sponge Nevus

C. Leukoedema
D. Leukoplakia

110. Which of the following is incorrect about Wheal?
A. It results due to short lived vasoconstriction
B. It results due to change in the flow of circulation to the site
C. It results due to an inflammatory response
D. It results due to vasopermeablity change

111. A 50-Year-old male patient, complained of single painful ulcer in Hard palate with productive cough since 6 months. It is provisionally diagnosed as
A. Pemphigus
B. Gumma
C. Squamous cell carcinoma
D. Tuberculosis

112. Aspirin, when prescribed as an analgesic; it is contraindicated in all of the following given conditions, *except*
A. Hypertension
B. Pregnancy
C. Peptic Ulcer
D. Bronchial Asthma

113. A 65-Year-old male patient reports with a single, deep looking ulcer present in the posterior hard palate since 1 week. It shows no signs of healing till now. On questioning, patient gives a negative history of tobacco or alcohol abuse and non-contributory medical and drug history. What is the provisional diagnosis?
A. Squamous cell carcinoma
B. Necrotizing sialometaplasia
C. Tuberculosis
D. Mucormycosis

114. Oral Corticosteroids are considered to have superior anti-inflammatory properties in comparison to Non-steroidal anti-inflammatory drugs, by virtue of:
    A. Their mode of action – by Blocking COX 2 enzyme only
    B. Their mode of action – by Block both COX 1 & 2 Enzyme
    C. Their mode of action – by Block Phospholipase A2
    D. Their mode of action is concentrated only in higher centers

115. As per the biomechanics of TMJ, while opening the jaw, there are two movements which the condyle will exhibit, namely Rotational and translation respectively. After an initial rotation movement on slight opening of jaw, which of the following Ligament which restrict further rotational movement of TMJ?
    A. Sphenomandibular Ligament
    B. Transverse fibers of Lateral Ligament
    C. Oblique Fibers of Lateral Ligament
    D. Stylomandibular Ligament

116. In a healthy individual, which of the following biochemical process is upregulated by insulin?
    A. Gluconeogenesis
    B. Glycolysis
    C. Glycogenesis
    D. Glycogenolysis

117. A teenage female reports to the dental clinic with complaint of multiple shallow ulcers in labial mucosa and alveolar mucosa with no signs similar cutaneous lesions. On questioning, she gives history of similar lesions last month. Incisional biopsy, gave a picture of non-specific inflammatory lesion. The provisional diagnosis is?
    A. Pemphigus
    B. Secondary Herpes Simplex
    C. Erythema Multiforme
    D. Minor Recurrent Aphthous Ulcer

118. A 30-year-old female patient reports with the complaint of intermittent swelling and recurrent pus discharge from the pre-maxillary area since 2 years. On questioning, she didn't reveal any history of trauma to the maxillary anterior teeth and even on clinical examination, no sign of pulp necrosis was seen. Shallow periodontal pockets were found on probing. On Perapical radiograph, a well-defined radiolucency is seen with corticated borders, intervening between anterior nasal spine. Provisional diagnosis is:
    A. Nasopalatine duct cyst
    B. Periodontal Cyst
    C. Stafne's Bone cyst
    D. Globulomaxillary cyst

119. A male patient reported with a slow growing, white colored, small, rough-surfaced, pedunculated enlargement seen on the right buccal mucosa. On palpation it is firm in consistency. On further questioning, he confirmed a similar lesion in his genital organs. The condition is provisionally diagnosed as?
    A. Verruca Vulgaris
    B. Pyogenic Granuloma
    C. Condyloma Acuminatum
    D. Squamous Papilloma

120. A patient reported with a small, roughly oval, smooth surfaced swelling of about 1 × 2 cm in size seen in the mandibular posterior vestibular region since 6 months. On examination, a large grossly decayed tooth is seen in the same region, associated with chronic draining sinus. The swelling is mild tender and firm on palpation. The condition is provisionally diagnosed as?
    A. EpulisFissuratum
    B. Traumatic Fibroma
    C. Parulis
    D. Pulp Polyp

REFERENCES

Burket's Oral Medicine (11th Ed.), BC Decker Inc., Canada.

Coleman, GC; Nelson, JF. *Principles of Oral Diagnosis.*, 1992, Mosby-Year Book.

Hutchinson's Clinical Methods (21st Ed.), Saunders, London.

Kerr, DA; Ash, M; Millard, MHD. *Oral diagnosis.*, 3rd ed. Saint Louis: Mosby Co.

Little, JW; Miller, C; Rhodus, NL. *Little and Falace's Dental Management of the Medically Compromised Patient.*, 2017, 9th Ed. Mosby.

Okeson, J. *Management of Temporomandibular Disorders and Occlusion.*, 2012; 7th Ed. Mosby.

Scully, C. *Scully's Medical Problems in Dentistry.*, 2014, 7th Ed. Churchil Livingstone.

Shafer's Textbook of Oral Pathology (6th Ed.), Elsevier, India.

Wood, NK; Goaz, PW. *Differential Diagnosis of Oral and Maxillofacial Lesions.*, 1997, 5th Ed. Mosby.

In: Scenario Based MCQ in Dentistry ISBN: 978-1-53617-298-0
Editors: M. Khursheed Alam et al.

Chapter 2

SCENARIO BASED MCQS IN ORAL RADIOLOGY

Santosh Patil, MDS, Anil Kumar, MDS, Radhika Doppalapudi, MDS and Shaliputra Magar, MDS
Oral Radiology, Oral Surgery Department,
College of Dentistry, Jouf University, Aljouf, Saudi Arabia

Radiology is a science dealing with x-rays and their applications in diagnosis and treatment of diseases. Oral and maxillofacial Radiology deals especially with imaging in relation to oral, dental and craniofacial diseases. It includes radiation physics (principles of x-ray production), radiation biology, radiation protection from primary and secondary radiation, intra oral periapical techniques, localization of radiographic techniques, anatomical landmarks of the teeth and jaws. It also deals with extra oral imaging techniques like panoramic radiography, cephalometric imaging and TMJ imaging which help in diagnosing the fractures of facial skeleton and malocclusion as well as during the entire treatment of these patients. The radiographic appearances of radiolucent, radiopaque and mixed lesions of the craniofacial region pave the way in differentiating the lesions for an appropriate diagnosis. Digital radiology had unique advantages in orthognathic surgeries, endodontics and delineating the cysts and tumors of head and neck region. The advances in implant imaging helps in ideal placement of implants. Contrast radiography in salivary gland helps in diagnosing salivary gland diseases. Apart from all these, the applied principles of radiotherapy help in management of head and neck cancers. These MCQs help the dental student's and also the practitioners in understanding and to gain the knowledge of radiation physics, biology, techniques, safety concerns and fundamentals of radiographic interpretation.

1. Which is a property of electromagnetic waves?
   A. Cause ionization
   B. Have mass and weight
   C. Travel at the velocity of light in vacuum
   D. Do not cause biologic changes in living cells

2. Which component of the X-ray machine is necessary in order to generate and accelerate electrons?
   A. Focal spot
   B. Power supply
   C. Tube vacuum
   D. Focusing cup

3. Doubling the exposure time will result in which occurrence?
   A. Doubling the range of photon energies
   B. Doubling the number of photons generated
   C. Decreasing by half the x-ray emission spectrum
   D. Decreasing by half the number of electrons produced

4. Which statement best describes a direct effect of radiation
   A. Action of radiation on water
   B. Formation of free radicals by biologic molecules

C. Loss of radiosensitive ells, affecting function of organ
D. Interaction of hydrogen and hydroxyl free radicals with organic molecules

5. Which is the recommended treatment to regain function of the muscles of mastication after radiation –caused inflammation and fibrosis?
   A. Antibiotics
   B. Exercise program
   C. Cessation of radiotherapy
   D. Restriction in mouth opening

6. The higher rate of cell division and differentiation of hematopoietic stem cells accounts for higher incidences of:
   A. Cataracts
   B. Leukemia
   C. Solid tumors
   D. Thyroid cancers

7. Which is the allowed whole-body radiation exposure for occupationally exposed workers?
   A. 1 mSv annual effective dose
   B. 50 mSv annually
   C. 100 mSv in a 5-year cumulative effect
   D. 150 mSv lifelong

8. The effective dose of radiation received by a patient who receives an FMX with F-speed film and round collimation is about 171μSv or the equivalent of how many days of background exposure?
   A. 0.6
   B. 4
   C. 21
   D. 47

9. A planned activity to ensure consistent production of superior images with minimum patient and personnel exposure is called:
   A. Quality assurance
   B. Risk reduction training
   C. Radiation safety practice
   D. Principles of justification and optimization

10. What is the purpose of the layer of scintillating material coated on the charge coupled device (CCD) surface?
   A. Decrease sensitivity to white light
   B. Increase x-ray absorption efficiency
   C. Enhance production of electron-hole pairs
   D. Transfer each row of pixel charges to the next row

11. Which is the advantage of CCD/CMOS dental imaging over PSP dental imaging?
   A. Programmed processor
   B. Plates loaded on drum system
   C. Dim light environment desirable
   D. Immediate image acquisition and display

12. The DIACOM standard recognizes which of the following?
   A. Privatization of image formats
   B. Need to export and import images effectively
   C. Necessity of sharing information between imaging devices
   D. Adaptation of developed technologies according to individual needs

13. Which film type contains silver halide grains that are flat, tabular crystals about 1.8 μm diameter?
   A. InSight
   B. Panoramic
   C. Duplicating
   D. Ultra-Speed

14. What is the purpose of green dyes added to the surface of the silver halide grains?
    A. Decrease film fog
    B. Take advantage of crossover light
    C. Increase light-absorbing capability
    D. Compensate for machine movement

15. Which best explains the importance of matching green-emitting screens with green sensitive films and blue–emitting screens with blue-sensitive films?
    A. Varying sizes of films and cassettes
    B. Color coordination enhances image sharpness
    C. Manufacturers' specifications prevent interchangeability
    D. Different phosphors fluoresce in different portions of the spectrum

16. A radiographic image with few shades of gray is said to have:
    A. Low contrast
    B. High contrast
    C. Long scale contrast
    D. Black-white contrast

17. Which phenomenon is responsible for enlargement of the radiographic image?
    A. Practitioner's skill
    B. Divergent paths of photons
    C. Object-to-receptor distance
    D. Increased number of electrons produced

18. To minimize distortion, which is the ideal position of the image receptor in relationship to the object?
    A. Perpendicular to the beam
    B. At right angles to the object
    C. Parallel to the long axis of the object
    D. As far from the object as structurally possible

19. If the central ray is directed at an angle that is inclined with more negative angulation to the bisector, the resulting image is
    - A. Magnified
    - **B. Elongated**
    - C. Proportional
    - D. Foreshortened

20. Which landmark is used to establish the proper horizontal angulation for premolar images?
    - A. Distal half of canine
    - **B. Buccal plane of premolars**
    - C. Long axis of premolar teeth
    - D. Mesial interproximal area of first molar

21. The parameter of CBCT that determines the number of shades of gray available to display the attenuation is called the
    - **A. Bit depth**
    - B. Frame rate
    - C. Scan volume
    - D. Spatial resolution

22. Which is a low-grade inflammation of the bone that appears as a radiopaque area extending below the roots of the tooth?
    - A. Pericoronitis
    - **B. Osteomyelitis**
    - C. Idiopathic resorption
    - D. Periapical inflammatory lesion

23. All are radiographic features of the keratocystic odontogenic tumor (KOT) *except* one, which one is the EXCEPTION?
    - A. Most common location is the posterior body of the mandible
    - B. Shows evidence of a cortical border, when not secondarily infected
    - **C. Internal structure is most commonly radiopaque**
    - D. Curved internal septa may be present

24. Torus palatinus, torus mandibularis, and dense bone island are examples of
    A. Hyperostosis
    B. Benign tumors
    C. Buccal exostoses
    D. Odontogenic organization

25. Which condition should be suspected if there are five or more dense bone islands (DBI) present radiographically?
    A. Peutz-Jeghers syndrome
    B. Hyperexostoses
    C. Ostogenic sarcoma
    D. Gardner's syndrome

26. Oral lesions of Langerhans' cell histiocytosis
    A. Form slowly over many years
    B. Cause sharp transient pain
    C. Produce bony swelling
    D. Occur in 90% of documented cases of Langerhans'

27. Edentulous patients with Paget's disease may experience which complication?
    A. Tight, poorly fitting dentures
    B. Sensitivity to denture materials
    C. Denture-induced fungal infections
    D. Exostosis removal for denture fabrication

28. Which is the most common cancer discovered on oral examination?
    A. Sarcoma
    B. Carcinoma
    C. Metastatic lesions from distant sites
    D. Malignancies of hematopoietic system

29. Which rarely occurs with non-Hodgkin's lymphoma?
    A. Pruritus
    B. Mobile teeth
    C. Lymphadenopathy
    D. Reactive bone formation

30. Which is the most common radiographic manifestation of progressive systemic sclerosis?
    A. General osteoporosis
    B. Large, coarse trabeculae
    C. Increased PDL space
    D. Enlarged and protruded maxillary alveolar ridge.

31. 33-year-old male patient comes to clinic with slow growing swelling in angle of mandible. Radiograph shows radio-opaque lesion with radiolucent border. What's your diagnosis?
    A. Osteosarcoma
    B. Osteoma.
    C. Fibrous dysplasia
    D. Cementoblastoma

32. A 20-year female patient's radiograph shows a radiolucent area surrounding the apices of mandibular anterior teeth which are vital. The most probable diagnosis is
    A. Periapical abscess
    B. Periapical granuloma
    C. Periapical cemental dysplasia
    D. Condensing osteitis

33. A 60-year-old male report for denture adjustment. His OPG shows 1 cm lytic area in the lower bicuspid region. The most probable diagnosis is
    A. Residual cyst
    B. Hyperparathyrodism

C. Carcinoma prostate

D. Any one of the above

34. Patient came with chief complaint of reddish discoloration of maxillary left central incisor, had a history of trauma. The periapical radiograph shows small radioluceny in the pulp chamber. It could be
    A. Interproximal bone loss.
    B. Internal resorption
    C. Radiopacity in the pulp chamber
    D. Rarefaction of radiograph

35. A patient has radiolucent lesion in the posterior mandible, anterior to the angle, has radiographic features of a cyst. After surgery, the histology report shows submaxillary salivary gland tissues. The lesion is likely
    A. Residual cyst
    B. Traumatic bone cyst
    C. Stafne's bone cyst
    D. Dentigerous cyst

36. OPG shows multiple radiopacities. What will be your Radiological interpretation?
    A. Multiple myeloma
    B. Cherubism
    C. Osteopetrosis
    D. Odontomas

37. Radiologically, a characteristic unilocular radiolucency seen in all of the following *except*
    A. Ameloblastoma
    B. Primodial cyst
    C. Giant cell granuloma
    D. Calcifyfing epithelial odontogenic tumor

38. Male patient visited the dental clinic following road traffic accident. If you are suspecting a bilateral condylar fracture, the best projection that would be preferred would be
    A. Occiptomental
    B. Reverse town
    C. Lateral Oblique 30 degree
    D. Panoramic

39. A female patient visits a dental clinic with a swelling in the mandible posterior region. On clinical examination 3rd molar was missing and on radiologic examination, a pericoronal radiolucency was noticed. The most likely diagnosis would be
    A. Odontogenic Keratocyst
    B. Radicular cyst
    C. Central cyst
    D. Dentigerous cyst

40. Patient complains of swelling in submandibular region, swelling increases before and during eating process, which type of X-ray used for diagnosis
    A. Occlusal radiograph
    B. Panoramic radiograph
    C. Sialography
    D. Angiograhy

41. A 30-year-old male patient reported with deep caries in the lower molar, no symptoms and there is radiopaque lesion at the apex of the distal root of the tooth. It could be
    A. Condensing osteitis
    B. Periapical granuloma
    C. Cemental dysplasia
    D. Periapical cyst

42. Among the following which extraoral radiograph best demonstrates the subcondylar fracture?
    A. Reverse Towne projection
    B. Anterior-posterior mandible
    C. Submentovertex
    D. Occipitomental

43. Which radiographic method you will suggest to check TMJ range of movement?
    A. Cranial Imagery
    B. Transcranial view
    C. Computerized tomography
    D. Arthography

44. A pregnant lady in her third trimester visited the dental clinic with the chief complaint of severe pain in maxillary molar tooth indicated for endodontic treatment. One should make a radiograph or not?
    A. Strictly contraindicated
    B. Less exposure time radiograph
    C. High sensitive film
    D. Perform radiograph with Lead apron & thyroid collar

45. A 32 year old male patient reported pain in TMJ and extra auricular region, On panoramic radiograph, what significant finding suggestive of Eagle‘s syndrome?
    A. Elongation of sphenoid process
    B. **Elongation of styloid process**
    C. Elongation of sphenoid and styloid process
    D. None of above

46. Patient with TMJ pain, TMJ ankylosis and generalized hypercementosis. On radiographic examination, bony pattern shows cotton-wool appearance. What will be your Diagnosis?
    A. Hyperparathyroidism
    B. Mono-ostotic fibrous dysplasia
    C. Paget's disease
    D. Cushing syndrome

47. Young patient came with the complaint of discoloration of right upper anterior. On vitality test, there was a negative response. On an X-ray a radiolucent lesion of diameter of about 2 cm with radiopaque lining was noticed. Which type of cyst it would be?
    A. Dentigerous cyst
    B. Lateral periodontal cyst
    C. Radicular cyst
    D. Residual cyst

48. An oval shaped radiolucent area is seen on OPG between the apices of maxillary central incisors. Which of the following normal anatomical landmarks could it be?
    A. **Nasopalatine foramen**
    B. Lingual foramen
    C. Nasal fossa
    D. Incisive canal

49. Which of the following help in distinguishing an osseous neoplasm and a cyst on x ray?
    A. Size.
    B. Shape.
    C. Location
    D. Content of the lesion

50. All the following lesions showing radiolucency on a radiograph *except*
    A. Ameloblastoma
    B. Cementoblastoma

C. Keratocyst
D. Central giant cell granuloma

51. What is the characteristic radiographic feature of Osteosarcoma?
A. Distinct sclerotic borders
B. Geographic bone destruction
C. Sunburst appearance
D. Radiolucent lesion

52. Patient visits a dental clinic with a complaint of swelling in mandibular region. On a radiograph, it showed onion peel appearance of bone. The patient is suffering from hyperthyroidism and hyperpigmentation of skin was noted. What would be the condition of?
A. Garre's osteomyelitis
B. Ewing's sarcoma
C. Osteogenic Carcinoma
D. Fibrous dysplasia

53. In the radiographic principle, "SLOB rule," same side movement of the object is ______ and the opposite side movement of the object is ______. What are the missing words in the same sequence?
A. Lateral and buccal
B. Lingual and buccal
C. Lingual and both sides
D. Lateral and both sides

54. All of the following are types of particulate radiation *except*
A. Alpha particle
B. Beta particle
C. Protons
D. **Nucleons**

55. A patient requires tooth extraction from an area that has been subjected to radiation therapy. Which of the following represents the greatest danger to this patient?
    A. Garre's osteomyelitis
    B. Ewing's sarcoma
    C. **Osteoradionecrosis**
    D. Fracture of mandible

56. Patient had decay of enamel following after radiotherapy. It could be due to
    A. Decrease in salivary flow
    B. Direct radiation contacting the enamel
    C. Desiccation of tooth structure
    D. Hypocalcification and pitting of enamel

57. Patient visited to the dental clinic complaining of pain and patient unable to tell the origin of pain. Upon examination even you can't find a clue. What are the next logical steps you will do in investigation?
    A. Multiple Intraoral radiograph
    B. Panoramic radiograph
    C. CT scan
    D. MRI

58. The X-ray shows tennis racket radiopaque lines of the posterior mandible. The diagnosis will be
    A. Garre's syndrome
    B. Osteosarcoma
    C. Fibrous dysplasia
    D. Odotogenic myxoma

59. Which type of radiograph shows condylar head orientation and facial Asymmetry?
    A. Reverse Towne
    B. Transorbital

C. Orthopantomography (OPG)
D. Submentovertex

60. The radiograph frequently used in Orthodontics for study of the growth and development of the head is
   A. AP Skull
   B. PA Skull
   C. Lateral Cephalometric view
   D. Panoramic view

61. A 25-year-old patient met with an accident and presented with a swelling on the right side of the face and he was unable to move the mandible laterally. The radiographic examination would include which of the following
   A. Intraoral periapical radiograph
   B. Occlusal radiograph
   C. Lower 90 occlusal radiograph
   D. Panoramic radiograph

62. During preoperative treatment planning of an implant in edentulous mandible, panoramic radiography provides information on
   A. Buccolingual width of mandible
   B. Depth of submandibular fossa
   C. Position of inferior alveolar canal
   D. The extent of the maxillary antra

63. A 28-year-old male patient had an edentulous space in the left first molar region. Following placement of implants, the post-operative radiographic evaluation of implant is recommended using
   A. Bisecting angle technique periapical radiograph
   B. CT
   C. Paralleling angle technique periapical radiograph
   D. MRI

64. A panoramic radiograph of a 5-year-old boy is depicting bilateral well defined multilocular lesions affecting the mandible. The probable diagnosis is
    A. Fibrous dysplasia
    B. Cherubism
    C. Odontogenic fibroma
    D. Focal osseous dysplasia

65. Panoramic radiograph in a patient is showing altered trabecular pattern in both maxilla and mandible with thinning of lower border of mandible with obliteration of the antra. In the same patient, true lateral skull is showing pronounced hair on end appearance with obliteration of antra. The probable diagnosis is
    A. Thalassemia
    B. Periapical osseous dysplasia
    C. Focal osseous dysplasia
    D. Florid osseous dysplasia

66. In a 30-year-old male patient, periapical radiograph is showing typical radiopaque mass at the apex of permanent first molar. The mass is attached to the root and has a thin radiolucent line around it. The probable diagnosis is
    A. Dentigerous cyst
    B. Odontogenic keratocyst
    C. Fibrous dysplasia
    D. Cementoblastoma

67. In a 34-year-old male patient, there was mild to moderate periodontitis. Panoramic radiograph is showing a round, well defined unilocular cyst-like appearance at the angle of mandible, below the inferior alveolar canal
    A. Stafne's bone cavity
    B. Fibrous dysplasia
    C. Periapical osseous dysplasia
    D. Ossifying fibroma

68. Panoramic radiograph is showing elongated calcified stylohyoid ligament and is a feature of
    A. Eagle's syndrome
    B. Crouzon's syndrome
    C. Apert syndrome
    D. Craniofacial dysostosis

69. A patient had a history of trauma 2 weeks back and on radiograph there is vertical root fracture. The patient is presenting with
    A. Erythema
    B. Pigmentation
    C. Both erythema and pigmentation
    D. Persistent low level dull pain.

70. A 32-year-old male patient came with pain and swelling in the floor of the mouth. Patient had severe pain while chewing food. Which radiograph do you suggest?
    A. IOPA
    B. Occlusal radiograph
    C. Paranasal sinus view
    D. Reverse Towne's view

71. A 20-year-old male patient came with a chief complaint of crowded teeth. On examination there were skeletal abnormalities and hypoplasia of mandible with angles class II anterior open bite. The probable associated diagnosis is
    A. Eagle's syndrome
    B. Treacher Collins syndrome
    C. Acromegaly
    D. Osteomyelitis

72. A 40-year-old female patient presented with localized cyst-like lesions within the jaws and long bones. There was generalized skeletal bone resorption. Loss of lamina dura of teeth is observed with ground glass appearance. The probable condition is
    A. Paget's disease
    B. Acromegaly
    C. Eagles syndrome
    D. Hyperparathyroidism

73. A 32-year-old patient had trauma and he is diagnosed as having a fracture of neck of the condyle. Which of the following view is favoring the diagnosis?
    A. PA skull
    B. 30°occipitomental view
    C. 0° occipitomental view
    D. Reverse Towne's view

74. A radiograph is depicting that there are two teeth which were joined together but arising from a single tooth germ, the condition is termed as
    A. Fusion
    B. Macrodontia
    C. Microdontia
    D. Gemination

75. Fracture of cranial base is better viewed in which of the following radiograph
    A. Panoramic radiograph
    B. PA view
    C. Submentovertex view
    D. Occipitomental view

76. In CBCT, Pixel and voxel represents cell in
    A. One and two dimensions
    B. Three and four dimensions
    C. Two and three dimensions
    D. Four and three dimensions

77. In a 25-year-old patient, a radiograph is made for an impacted tooth. Winters lines are drawn. Red line represents
    A. Line along occlusal surfaces of 1st& 2nd molars.
    B. Line along crest of interdental bone
    C. Margin of alveolar bone surrounding the tooth
    D. Point of application of elevator

78. In sialography, the sialographic appearance of tree in winter or leafless tree appearance is seen in
    A. Normal submandibular gland
    B. Normal parotid gland
    C. Sjogren's syndrome
    D. Sialedenitis

79. The main methods of localization of unerupted maxillary canines is
    A. Parallax in horizontal plane using two periapicals
    B. Parallax in horizontal plane using panoramic and occlusal
    C. Lower 90 occlusal
    D. Mandibular occlusal

80. Oblique lateral radiographs are taken using
    A. An extraoral cassette and a skull unit
    B. An extraoral cassette and a Cephalostat
    C. An extraoral cassette and a dental x-ray set
    D. A film packet and a Cephalostat

81. Photostimulable Phosphor plates consist of
    A. Silicon with scintillation layer
    B. Intensifying Screens below the silicon
    C. Barumflourohalide phosphor
    D. Complementary metal oxide semiconductors

82. In a 15-year-old male patient, a radiograph is depicting teeth with bulbous crowns, cervical constriction, short roots and obliteration of pulp chamber and root canals. The anomaly is
    A. Amelogenesis imperfecta
    B. Dentinogenesis imperfecta
    C. Dentin dysplasia
    D. Hypocalcified amelogenesis imperfecta

83. A 60-year-old female patient presented with swelling in anterior part of hard palate. Occlusal radiograph revealed large well-defined radiolucent lesion in maxilla. The probable diagnosis is
    A. Solitary bone cyst
    B. Osteosarcoma
    C. Metastatic tumor
    D. Nasopalatine duct cyst

84. A 65-year-old male patient is presenting with an ulcerative lesion in the floor of the mouth on the left side. Panoramic radiograph revealed ragged and infiltrative irregular borders involving the left mandible. The condition would be
    A. Hyperparathyroidism
    B. Aneurysmal bone cyst
    C. Malignancy involving bone
    D. Central ossifying fibroma

85. Which one of the following is a multilocular radiolucent lesion
    A. Lateral periodontal cyst
    B. Nasopalatine duct cyst
    C. Solitary bone cyst
    D. KCOT

86. A 50-year-old male patient is presenting with a painless bony swelling in the left body of mandible. To assess the buccolingual expansion of mandible which of the following view is taken
    A. Lower 90° occlusal
    B. Lower 45° occlusal
    C. Standard occipitomental view
    D. PA jaws

87. Paranasal sinus view revealed well defined homogenous radiopacity in the maxillary sinus. The condition could be due to
    A. Rhinolith
    B. Antrolith
    C. Phlebolith
    D. Sialolith

88. A 30-year-old male patient reported with mobility of teeth and bleeding from gingiva. Clinical examination revealed rebound mobility of teeth. Radiograph showed sun ray appearance and serpegenous enlargement of mandibular canal. What could be this lesion?
    A. Neurofibroma
    B. Hemangioma
    C. Ameloblastoma
    D. Fibrous dysplasia

89. An 18-year-old female reported with a chief complaint of missing maxillary anterior tooth. Patient informed that permanent teeth in that region did not erupt after exfoliation of deciduous teeth. Intraoral examination revealed missing permanent maxillary right canine. Maxillary occlusal radiograph showed impacted maxillary canine. Along with this multiple miniature tooth-like structures of varying densities were present pericoronal to the impacted canine. What could be this lesion?
    A. Compound odontome
    B. Ameloblastoma
    C. AOT
    D. CEOT

90. A 25-year old male patient reported with the missing maxillary canine. On a periapical radiograph, a well-defined radiolucency with the borders attached to the CEJ of the impacted canine was noticed. The most probable diagnosis could be
    A. Odontogenic Keratocyst/Keratocystic Odontogenic tumor
    B. Ameloblastoma
    C. Nasopalatine cyst
    D. Dentigerous cyst

91. While extracting maxillary second premolar, you suspect that root is displaced into maxillary sinus. So which radiograph is best in this case?
    A. Panoramic radiograph
    B. Lateral Cephalogram
    C. Occlusal radiograph
    D. Bitewing radiograph

92. A 25-year old female patient reported with the painful swelling in the anterior region of the palate. You make a periapical radiograph which shows a well-defined heart shaped radiolucency between maxillary central incisors. What could be this lesion?
    A. Odontogenic Keratocyst/KeratocysticOdontogenic tumor
    B. Ameloblastoma

C. Nasopalatine cyst
D. Dentigerous cyst

93. A 30-year old female patient reported with impacted mandibular third molar and limited mouth opening and on a panoramic radiograph which shows a well-defined multilocular radiolucency with scalloped border in the third molar and ramus region. The possible diagnosis could be
    A. Odontogenic Keratocyst/Keratocystic Odontogenic tumor
    B. Ameloblastoma
    C. Pindborg's tumor
    D. Dentigerous cyst

94. A 45-year old male patient reported with the large swelling on the left side of face. It was non tender and firm to hard in consistency. You make a panoramic radiograph which shows well defined multilocular honey comb radiolucency with corticated border in the third molar and ramus region. What could be this lesion?
    A. Fibrous dysplasia
    B. Ameloblastoma
    C. Pindborg's tumor
    D. Dentigerous cyst

95. A 25-year-old male patient came with a complaint of pain in the lower left back tooth region for a period of 5 days. Pain was recurrent in nature. There was history of an increase of the swelling during meals. Clinical examination revealed a firm, tender swelling on the floor of the mouth on the left side. Radiographic examination revealed two tubular radiopacities in the left side. What is your probable diagnosis?
    A. Submandibular tumor
    B. Lymphoma
    C. Lieomyoma
    D. Silaolithiasis

96. A 33-year-old female presented with throbbing right maxillary pain and swelling over the mid palatal region since 3 months. Patient gave a history of trauma to the upper front teeth during his childhood. On clinical examination, a mid-palatal swelling was found which was firm in consistency non tender. Maxillary right central incisor was discoloured and non-vital. Radiographic examination revealed a well-defined radiolucency around the central incisor. What is your provisional diagnosis?
    A. Minor salivary gland tumor
    B. Lymphoma
    C. Liopma
    D. Radicular cyst

97. A 15-year-old female patient presented with a swelling on her upper left jaw in the region of the front teeth since a year. Intra-oral examination, a single, well-circumscribed radiolucency was present in the labial and palatal aspect of the left upper anterior maxillary region. The permanent maxillary left lateral incisor and canine were missing. Radiographs revealed a well-circumscribed unilocular radiolucency in relation to the left maxillary incisor to first premolar region associated with an impacted left maxillary lateral incisor and canine with mesially displaced root of the left maxillary central incisor; in addition, specks of calcification in the radiolucent area were present. What is your provisional diagnosis?
    A. Adenomatoid odontogenic tumor
    B. Ameloblastoma
    C. Dentigerous cyst
    D. Radicular cyst

98. An 18-year-old female patient presented with a chief complaint of bony swelling at right lower back region of the jaw since 3 months. The swelling was ill defined extending from antero-posteriorly from the parasymphysis region till the angle of mandible. Panoramic view was showing ill-defined radio-opacity showing a ground glass

appearance involving lower border of the mandible extending up to alveolar ridge and superior displacement of mandibular canal. What is your provisional diagnosis?

A. Fibrous dysplasia
B. Ameloblastoma
C. Dentigerous cyst
D. Radicular cyst

99. An 8-year-old girl patient presented with slowly growing painless, bilaterally symmetrical swelling of the jaw. Enlargement involved whole jaw. Enlarged jaw was hard to palpate. Eyes were displaced superiorly. Orthopantamograph and antero-posterior view of skull radiograph revealed bilateral, multilocular, radiolucent lesion with thinning of cortical plates and displacement of unerupted teeth anteriorly in mandible. What is your provisional diagnosis?

A. Adenomatoid odontogenic tumor
B. Ameloblastoma
C. Dentigerous cyst
D. Cherubism

100. A 67-year-old female patient reported with s slow-progressive swelling in the lower jaw for past few years. Extra oral examination reveals broadening and widening of the lower facial view with thickened lower lip. Intra oral examination showed increased size and altered shape of the mandibular alveolar ridge, pseudo micrognathia of the maxillary arch and partially edentulous, thickened cortical plate. OPG shows hypercementosis with displacement of involved teeth, cortical thickening of the body of the mandible and cotton wool appearance on both sides of the mandible. What is your provisional diagnosis?

A. Fibrous dysplasia
B. Ameloblastoma
C. Cherubism
D. Paget's disease

101. A 36-year-old female patient reported with swelling over the right side of the lower jaw. Face was asymmetric with a diffuse swelling over the right side of the face. Third molar was clinically missing. . OPG showed a mixed radiopaque-radiolucent lesion on the right body of mandible with impacted third molar being displaced posteriorly and horizontally. What is your provisional diagnosis?

    A. Calcifying epithelial odontogenic tumor
    B. Ameloblastoma
    C. Dentigerous cyst
    D. Cherubism

102. According to the basic principles of the paralleling technique, the film is placed in the mouth _________________ to the long axis of the tooth being radiographed, and the central ray of the x-ray beam is directed _____________________ to the film and the long axis of the tooth.

    A. parallel; perpendicular
    B. parallel; parallel
    C. perpendicular; parallel
    D. perpendicular; perpendicular

103. A bitewing film helps the clinician with the diagnosis of: 1. Interproximal caries, 2. Periapical lesions, 3. Periodontal disease?

    A. 1 only
    B. 2 only
    C. 3 only
    D. 1 and 3

104. For which of the following anatomical situations would a panoramic film be the best choice for getting the most accurate diagnostic information?

    A. Impacted third molars
    B. Shallow palate

C. Ankyloglossia
D. Shallow floor of the mouth

105. Size 1 film is always positioned with the long portion of the film in a ____________ direction, and size 2 film is always positioned with the long portion of the film in a ________________ direction. Paralleling Technique.
    A. vertical; vertical
    B. horizontal; horizontal
    C. vertical; horizontal
    D. horizontal; vertical

106. Elongated images refer to images of the teeth that appear ____________. Elongation of images results from ______________ vertical angulation.
    A. too long; excessive
    B. too long; insufficient
    C. shortened; excessive
    D. shortened; insufficient

107. When the Frankfort Plane is tipped up when taking a panoramic film, the image obtained will show
    A. **a squared-off mandible and palate superimposed over the maxillary teeth**
    B. shortened mandibular incisors
    C. a V-shaped mandible
    D. wider and blurred anterior teeth

108. In which of the following anatomical variants would you most likely utilize a tongue blade to aid in taking the film?
    A. Tori
    B. Ankyloglossia
    C. Impacted third molars
    D. Shallow palate

109. There are several methods for obtaining radiographic information in a patient who has limited mouth opening due to trismus. Which of the following methods would be best?
    A. Periapical film with hemostat
    B. Occlusal film
    C. Panoramic film
    D. Lateral Cephalometry

110. Mr. Khalid presented with an OPG that reveals missing all four first premolars and all four third molars. The rest of the teeth are present (24 teeth). The teeth are all in contact, with no edentulous spaces. The majority of the teeth have extensive caries and/or restorations and you have decided to take periapical films of the entire mouth, along with posterior horizontal bitewings. (You will be using the paralleling technique with # 1 films anteriorly, # 2 films posteriorly). How many periapical films would be needed for Mr. Khalid?
    A. 9
    B. 10
    C. 11
    D. 13

111. The radiolucent lesion you have identified in the periapical region of the mandibular anterior teeth has a smooth, rounded periphery with well-defined corticated borders. There is no pain or swelling associated with this area. This lesion is most likely
    A. Inflammation
    B. Benign
    C. Malignant
    D. a and c

112. You are taking a maxillary molar periapical x-ray on a patient. Why would you normally use the paralleling technique instead of the bisecting angle technique?
    A. The film placement is more comfortable for the patient.

B. The exposure time will be less.
C. The film placement antero-posteriorly is not as critical.
D. There will usually be less distortion of the image.

113. Many patients are concerned about the potential adverse effects of ionizing radiation. Which of the following imaging techniques does not use ionizing radiation?
A. Sialography
B. Arthrography
C. CT
D. Ultrasound

114. A 30-year-old female patient reported with Polyostotic fibrous dysplasia, Melanotic skin pigmentation (Café-au-lait spots) and Precocious puberty. What could be this lesion?
A. Gardner's syndrome
B. Sjogren's syndrome
C. Steven Johnson syndrome
D. Albright's syndrome

115. A 47-year-old female patient reported with swelling in the lower jaw for past few years. History reveals a slow-progressive swelling. Examination showed increased size and altered shape of the mandibular alveolar ridge, pseudomicrognathia of the maxillary arch and partially edentulous, thickened cortical plate. Orthopantomograph shows ground glass, orange-peel and smoke-screen pattern. What is your provisional diagnosis?
A. Fibrous dysplasia
B. Ameloblastoma
C. Cherubism
D. Paget's disease

116. A 47-year-old female patient reported with hydrocephalus, blindness, deafness, vestibular nerve dysfunction, and facial paralysis. Orthopantomograph shows bilaterally symmetric increase in bone density. The entire bone was mildly enlarged. The difference between cortical and cancellous bone was not well appreciated. Because of the increased bone density, the roots of the teeth were not be apparent. What is your provisional diagnosis?
    A. Fibrous dysplasia
    B. Osteopetrosis
    C. Cherubim
    D. Paget's disease

117. Which is the least radiosensitive organ in the field of typical dental x-ray?
    A. Thyroid
    B. Bone marrow
    C. Lymphoid tissue
    D. Teeth

118. The amount of radiation required to produce a particular density is known as
    A. **Speed**
    B. Density
    C. Contrast
    D. Fog

119. The basic technology behind MRI is, that it is safe method of imaging as it uses
    A. Ionizing radiation
    B. Sound waves
    C. Electric waves
    D. **Magnetic energy**

120. Which radiographic view is considered the primary view for evaluating the alveolar bone in periodontal disease?
    A. Periapical
    B. OPG
    C. Bitewing
    D. Occlusal

121. Among the following, which imaging technique is the best to evaluate the soft tissue components of the temporomandibular joint?
    A. CBCT
    B. OPG
    C. MRI
    D. CT

122. Which radiograph shows clearly, the medial, lateral and inferior borders of the maxillary sinus?
    A. Periapical view
    B. OPG view
    C. Water's view
    D. Occlusal view

123. The technique in which, a radiopaque or contrast dye is injected through the duct openings into the salivary glands, is known as
    A. **Sialograph**y
    B. Arthrography
    C. Scintigraphy
    D. Angiography

124. You see on an OPG, a lesion which is above the mandibular canal and then you may consider that the lesion is....
    A. **Odontogenic origin**
    B. Non-odontogenic origin
    C. Salivary gland origin
    D. Epithelial origin

125. What is the most likely tissue of origin for a tumour in the mandibular canal?
   A. **Neurofibroma**
   B. Hemangioma
   C. Fibrous dysplasia
   D. Both a and b

126. What is the distance which is to be maintained while making radiograph?
   A. 2 feet
   B. 4 feet
   C. 6 feet
   D. 8 feet

127. Which of the following is not a usual radiographic signs of inflammatory disease involving the paranasal sinuses?
   A. Mucous membrane thickening
   B. Air-fluid levels
   C. Opacification of a sinus cavity
   D. Destruction of the cortical margins

128. When should bitewing views first be obtained for the typical child?
   A. After the eruption of primary molars
   B. After the eruption of permanent molars
   C. After eruption of permanent teeth on one side
   D. After the establishment of contacts on the posterior teeth.

129. There must be -----------% loss in mineralization before caries is radiographically evident with standard D- and E-speed intraoral films.
   A. 5-10%
   B. 10-20%
   C. 20-30%
   D. 30-60%

130. A foramen may be superimposed over the apices of teeth, mimicking the presence of periapical disease. What radiographic technique is most useful in distinguishing between normal structures and apical pathology?
    A. Tube shift technique
    B. Periapical technique
    C. Bitewing technique
    D. Occlusal technique

131. What is the earliest radiographic sign of periapical disease of pulpal origin?
    A. Widening of the periodontal ligament space
    B. Loss of interdental bone
    C. Periapical radiolucency
    D. Periapical radiopacity

132. What is the radiographic sign of an ankylosed tooth?
    A. Widening of the periodontal ligament space
    B. Loss of the periodontal ligament space and lamina aura
    C. Periapical radiolucency
    D. Periapical radiopacity

133. What is the diagnosis for a patient who has all his teeth with pulp that are reduced in size which is seen on an OPG?
    A. Dentinogenesis imperfecta
    B. Amelogenesis imperfecta
    C. Dentin dysplasia
    D. Congenital syphilis

134. An OPG shows all the teeth with generalized large pulp chambers, which of the following condition is you may think of?
    A. Hypoparathyroidism
    B. Hyperparathyroidism
    C. Hyperphosphotasia
    D. Cretinism

135. An OPG shows periosteal reaction, cloacae, sequestra and involucrum formation, what is your probable diagnosis?
    A. Abscess
    B. Osteomyelitis
    C. Cyst
    D. Tumor

136. The fracture of zygomatic arches are best examined with a
    A. Submentovertex view
    B. Waters view
    C. OPG
    D. Lateral Cephalometry

137. Which lesion does not commonly present as a soap-bubble or honeycomb appearance?
    A. Ameloblastoma
    B. Haemangioma
    C. Cherubism
    D. Fibrous dysplasia

138. What is the second most common radiographic sign of periapical disease of pulpal origin?
    A. Widening of the periodontal ligament space
    B. Loss of interdental bone
    C. Periapical radiolucency
    D. Loss of the lamina dura around the apex of the tooth

REFERENCES

Eric Whaites (2013). *Essentials of Dental Radiography and Radiology*, 5th Edition.

Langlais RP, Miller C. *Exercises in Oral Radiology and Interpretation.* 2017; 5th Ed. Saunders.

Langland OE, Langlais RP. *Principles of Dental Imaging*. 2002; 2nd Ed. lippincott williams & wilkins.

White and Pharoah (2014). *Oral Radiology principles and Interpretation,* 7th Edition.

Wood NK, Goaz PW. D*ifferential Diagnosis of Oral and Maxillofacial Lesions*. 1997; 5th Ed. Mosby.

In: Scenario Based MCQ in Dentistry ISBN: 978-1-53617-298-0
Editors: M. Khursheed Alam et al.

Chapter 3

SCENARIO BASED MCQS IN ORAL SURGERY

Arun Priya Srinivasan, Namdeo Prabhu and Mohamed Kassab
Oral Surgery, College of Dentistry,
Jouf University, Aljouf, Saudi Arabia

Oral and Maxillofacial surgery is a branch of dentistry, under the broad specialty of Oral-Maxillofacial surgery and diagnostic sciences, which deals with the complex treatment of the face, jaws and the oral cavity which primarily includes the surgical management, but also involves complex medical regimes which sometimes extend in the neck region. Oral and Maxillofacial surgery also deals with the diseases and defects that affect the Head and Neck region. Numbers of sub-specialties have evolved over the period of time which can be broadly classified as Oncosurgery, Plastic Reconstructive and Orthognathic surgery, TMJ surgery and Head and Neck Trauma. Apart from the surgical treatment, Pain management and Anesthesia also forms an important part of this field of dentistry, which amounts to medical and surgical management to treat any amount of pain which also sometimes includes those of neuronal origin like Neuralgias. At the simplest methods like Dental extraction and

Disimpaction of the teeth and alike tissue, along with cyst enucleation and debridement of the infection, it extends till the surgical resection of the cancer tissue and reconstruction of the missing parts of the Oral cavity and the face. A truly complex field, this branch of the dentistry is rightly addressed as a bridging link between the Surgery, Dentistry and Medicine which also encompasses the Anesthetic part.

The MCQs aid the student's and the practitioners to understand the subject effectively and to assess the knowledge acquired.

1. A 60-year-old patient suffered injuries to his lower half of face that suggested mandibular body fracture on examination. What is the most appropriate way of management of such a Patient where there is no presence of teeth?
   A. Gunning splint
   B. Cap splint
   C. Ribbon splint
   D. All of the above

2. Long term effect of radiotherapy to oral mucosa is characterized by
   A. Epithelium becomes more keratinized
   B. Sub mucosa becomes highly vascular
   C. Break down & delayed healing, submucosa less vascular
   D. No sub mucosal fibrosis

3. A 20-year-old patient met with a bike accident and CT scan revealed a displaced, unfavorable fracture in the mandibular angle region. During surgery it was seen that it was a fairly difficult fracture to treat? This might be because of
   A. Injury to neurovascular bundle
   B. Malocclusion secondary to injury
   C. Distraction of fracture segments by muscle pull
   D. Increased density of bone in this region of mandible

4. Any trauma sustained by a jaw bone and communicating with the teeth bearing section of the alveolus should be considered a
    A. Simple
    B. Open
    C. Greenstick
    D. Comminuted

5. An 8-year-old child was diagnosed with fracture in twin jaws and it was further noticed it was just a single fracture line. What is the best way of treating such a fracture?
    A. Cap splint fixation
    B. Intermaxillary fixation
    C. Risdon wiring
    D. Transosseous wiring

6. A patient came with history of sharp, lancinating pain on right side of face, not relieved by analgesics. On progressive symptoms carbamazepine was found to be effective in this patient. What is the most probable diagnosis?
    A. Acute pulpitis.
    B. Trigeminal neuralgia
    C. Acute dental abscess
    D. Dry socket

7. Any patient being instilled with cancer chemotherapy is candidate of myelosuppression, what is the most common manifestation of this?
    A. Anemia & thrombocytopenia
    B. Thrombocytosis
    C. Leukocytosis
    D. Lymphocytosis

8. All patients sustaining mandibular fracture will show one or all of the symptoms *except*
   A. Malocclusion
   B. Paresthesia of lower lip
   C. Fractured ends are prevented from dislocation by masticatory muscles
   D. Are usually compound

9. A 47-year-old patient was suffering from severe headache and heaviness of face since 4 days. On further evaluation it was noticed that there was inflammation of most or all of the paranasal sinuses simultaneously. This condition is best described as
   A. Pan sinusitis
   B. Sinusitis
   C. Paranasal sinusitis
   D. Parasinusitis

10. Most common culprit for Maxillary sinus infection of odontogenic origin is due to
   A. Aerobic bacteria
   B. Anaerobic bacteria
   C. Fungal
   D. Viral

11. During a peripheral posting in a hospital it was found out that there were only basic instruments available for treatment and no means of open reduction for treating facial skeleton was available. In such a scenario all of the following are the techniques can be of help *except*
   A. Risdon's wiring technique
   B. Eyelet wiring technique
   C. Erich's arch bar fixation
   D. Champy miniplates osteosynthesis

12. On doing a CT scan it was seen that mandible of a patient was badly comminuted and all fragments were grossly displaced due to muscle pull. Each of the muscle mentioned will cause displacement of the muscles *except* one. Which is that muscle?
    A. Lateral Pterygoid
    B. Medial Pterygoid
    C. Masseter
    D. Buccinator

13. During extraction of 16 and 17 root stump was broken and surgical procedure was instilled to remove the roots, but as soon as the root was retrieved, bubbling for the socket was seen and communication with the maxillary sinus was inferred. What is the best treatment for the accidental Oro-antral communication like this one during extraction which is around 0.5 mm in size?
    A. Buccal flap technique
    B. Palatal flap technique
    C. Periodic observation and follow up
    D. Caldwcll-luc approach

14. In WINTER'S classification, white line tells us
    A. Depth of the impacted tooth
    B. Angulation of the impacted tooth
    C. Point of application for elevator
    D. Used to classify fracture of the tooth

15. Various anatomical structures can involve in various levels of the facial trauma. In which of the following maxillary sinus is usually involved in fractures?
    A. Lefort 1
    B. Zygomatic arch fracture
    C. Lefort 3
    D. Nasoethmiodal fracture

16. Which of the following methods of sterilization is not as effective as other techniques?
    A. Ethylene oxide gas
    B. Gamma radiation
    C. UV radiation
    D. Autoclaving

17. If a patient comes with a history of cardiac problem taking aspirin what will be the possible complication if you do extraction
    A. Increases bleeding time
    B. Increases prothrombin time
    C. Increases clotting time
    D. Increases partial thrombin time

18. Cross bar elevator and winter-cryer works on mechanical principle of
    A. Wedge
    B. Lever
    C. Wheel & axle
    D. Pulley

19. While removing an impacted wisdom tooth, if we have to do the apicoectomy of 2nd molar also, which type of incision should be given?
    A. Semilunar
    B. Ward's
    C. Extended ward's
    D. Envelop

20. Which is the most commonly used size of suture in oral cavity
    A. 1/0
    B. 2/0
    C. 3/0
    D. 4/0

21. Which of the following can be said to have occurred if the patient develops severe pain on second postoperative day of mandibular 3rd molar disimpaction
    A. Hemorrhage
    B. Infection
    C. Dry socket
    D. Fracture of cortical plate

22. A 58-year-old man is attending surgery for extraction of his upper right canine and lateral incisor and his upper left second premolar and first molar, with insertion of an immediate partial denture. After extracting the teeth, you attempt to insert the denture but are unable to seat it. Which one of the following is the most likely cause of this problem?
    A. Bony undercut not blocked out
    B. Distortion of tissues by local anesthetic
    C. Failure to use a soft lining material
    D. Porosity introduced during processing of acrylic E Post-extraction swelling

23. A 45-year-old patient woke up with swollen face, puffiness around the eyes, and edema of the upper lip with redness and dryness. When he went to bed he had the swelling, pain or dental complaints. Examination shows several deep silicate restorations in the anterior teeth but examination is negative for caries, thermal tests, percussion, palpation, pain, and periapical area of rarefaction. The patient's temperature is normal. The day before he had a series of gastrointestinal x-rays at the local hospital and was given a clean bill of health. The condition is
    A. Acute periapical abscess
    B. Angioneurotic oedema
    C. Infectious mononucleosis
    D. Acute maxillary sinusitis

24. A 65-year-old woman arrived for dental therapy. The answered questionnaire shows that she is suffering from severe cirrhosis. The problem that can be anticipated in the routine dental therapy is
    A. Extreme susceptibility to pain
    B. Tendency towards prolonged hemorrhage
    C. Recurring oral infection
    D. Increased tendency to syncope

25. Patient received heavy blow to the right body of the mandible sustaining a fracture there. You should suspect a second fracture is most likely to be present in
    A. Symphysis region
    B. Left body of the mandible
    C. Left sub-condylar region
    D. Right sub-condylar region

26. Cardiac patient came to dental office which signs and symptoms that commonly suggest Cardiac failure in him being assessed for oral surgery are
    A. Elevated temperature and nausea
    B. Palpitations and malaise
    C. Ankle edema and dyspnea
    D. Erythema and pain

27. Patient with a cyst at the apex of an upper central incisor measuring 1 cm in diameter is visualized in radiograph and confirmed by aspiration biopsy; which method of treatment would you consider?
    A. Extraction of the central incisor and retrieving the cyst through the socket
    B. Exteriorizing the cyst through the buccal bone and mucosa
    C. Making a mucoperiosteal flap and removing the cyst through an opening made in the alveolar bone, followed by tooth removal

D. Making a mucoperiosteal flap and removing the cyst through an opening made in the alveolar bone, followed by endodontic treatment

28. A 40 year aged patient with a persistent oro-antral fistula for a 12 weeks period following the extraction of a maxillary first permanent molar is best treated by
    A. Further review and reassurance since it will most probably heal spontaneously
    B. Antibiotic therapy and nasal decongestants
    C. Curettage and dressing of the defect
    D. Excision of the fistula and surgical closure

29. A patient complains of a stomach upset 48 hours after starting a course of antibiotic for severe pericoronitis of lower right impacted wisdom tooth, this is an example of
    A. Type I allergic reaction
    B. Nervous disorder
    C. Side effect of the drug
    D. Type IV hypersensitivity reaction

30. A patient who is on long term aspirin therapy might show increased post-operative bleeding because aspirin inhibits
    A. Synthesis of thromboxane A_2 and prevents platelet aggregation
    B. Synthesis of prostacyclin and prevents platelet aggregation
    C. Synthesis of prostaglandin and prevents production of blood platelets
    D. Thrombin and prevents formation of the fibrin network

31. A patient who has been taking warfarin came to oral surgery for a procedure, which of the following is not true about warfarin
    - **A. INR of 3 is enough to start any extraction**
    - B. Affects extrinsic system and increases prothrombin time
    - C. Heparin can be given subcutaneously and acts rapidly
    - D. It takes at least 12 hours for Vitamin K to reverse the effects of coumarin

32. A 35 years old male patient came to oral surgery clinic with trigeminal neuralgia which of the following is NOT CHARACTERISTIC of trigeminal neuralgia?
    - A. The pain usually last for few seconds up to a minute in the early stages of the disease
    - B. The pain is usually unilateral
    - C. Patient characteristically have sites on the skin that when stimulated precipitate an attack of pain
    - **D. An attack of pain is usually preceded by sweating in the region of the forehead**

33. In a patient with impacted maxillary canine; by moving the X ray tube distally the canine moves distally too; where do you expect the impacted canine to be
    - A. Labially impacted
    - **B. Palatally impacted**
    - C. Lingually impacted
    - D. In the maxillary sinus

34. An 8-year-old child presents with all permanent incisors erupted, but yet only three permanent first molars are erupted. Oral examination revealed a large gingival bulge in the unerupted permanent molar area. A panoramic radiograph showed the alveolar emergence of the unerupted permanent first molar crown and three fourth root developments, there are no other radiographic abnormalities. The most appropriate diagnosis and treatment plan in such situation would be

A. Dentigerous cyst; surgical enucleation
B. Idiopathic failure of eruption, surgical soft tissues exposure
C. Ankylosis of the molar, removal of the first molar to allow the second one to erupt into its place
D. Ankylosis of the molar, surgical soft tissues exposure and luxation of the molar

35. A young patient of 24 years came with alveolar abscess related to upper right central incisor. What is the best treatment for alveolar abscess?
    A. Endodontic treatment or extraction
    B. Incision and drainage
    C. Extraction
    D. Endodontic treatment

36. A patient 58 years old came to oral surgeon with rheumatoid arthritis the most common complication of TMJ
    A. Ankylosis
    B. MPDS
    C. Internal derangement
    D. Osteoma of condyle

37. A patient came to hospital following an accident with bilateral parasymphyseal fractures of the mandible the segment is displaced posterior under influence of
    A. Anterior belly of Digastric muscle, Geniohyoid and Mylohyoid muscles
    B. Masseter, Lateral Pterygoid and Medial Pterygoid muscles
    C. Buccinator, anterior and posterior belly of Digastric muscle
    D. Geniohyoid, posterior belly of Digastric muscle and Genioglossus

38. Patient with lupus erythematosus and on cortisone needs a surgical extraction of a tooth. What should the surgeon instruct the patient?
    A. Take half of the cortisone dose at the day of operation
    B. Double the cortisone dose at the day of operation
    C. Take half of the cortisone dose day before and at the day of operation and day after
    D. Double the cortisone dose day before and at the day of operation and day after

39. Patient presents with lateral sub-conjunctival hemorrhage, infraorbital step & diplopia on right side with inability to open mouth. It could be
    A. Fracture subcondylar right side
    B. Fracture zygomatic right side
    C. Fracture Lefort II right side
    D. Fracture of the floor of the orbit

40. A patient presents bilateral infraorbital step, paraesthesia on left cheek region, with posterior gagging and mobility of maxillary complex at nasal bones. It indicates
    A. Bilateral fracture Zygomatic
    B. Bilateral fracture Lefort II
    C. Fracture Zygomatic left side with bilateral Lefort II
    D. Fracture bilateral sub condoyle & fracture Zygomatic left side

41. A 24-year- old patient presented with sub-conjunctival hemorrhage on medial & lateral side of eye & history of bleeding from nose and mouth with disturbed occlusion. On moving the maxilla, mobility was palpable at infraorbital margins only. It can be suspected to be fracture
    A. Lefort I
    B. Lefort II
    C. Lefort III
    D. Lefort II & fracture zygoma

42. A 58-year-old male patient complained of pain on right side of tongue, inability to protrude tongue, dysphagia, increased salivation & alteration in voice, one should suspect
    A. Carcinoma of anterior tongue
    B. Carcinoma of posterior tongue
    C. Carcinoma larynx
    D. Carcinoma epiglottis

43. A hypertension patient having café-au-lait spots, hypoplastic maxilla & signs of mental deficiency presented with soft tissue mass on buccal mucosa, this should incite surgeon to investigate for
    A. Neurofibromatosis
    B. Neurilemmoma
    C. Down syndrome
    D. Pierre Robion syndrome

44. If after extracting a mandibular tooth, one encounters bleeding due to an underlying haemangioma, the first step in treatment would be
    A. Carotid artery ligation
    B. Inferior alveolar artery ligation
    C. Replacing the tooth in the socket
    D. Pressure packing

45. A 12-year-old patient had episodes of haemarthrosis but characteristically petechiae & ecchymosis were not seen. His BT & platelet count was normal. It is hematological picture of
    A. Hemophilia A
    B. Thrombocytopenic purpura
    C. von Willebrand's disease
    D. Scurvy

46. A 12-year-old patient of thrombocytopenic purpura has to undergo minor oral surgery procedure; he should first be given
    A. Packed red cells to improve oxygen carrying capacity of blood
    B. Fresh frozen plasma to provide coagulation factors
    C. Platelet-rich plasma to allow normal clotting
    D. None of above since his BT/CT should be normal

47. Following roadside accident, a patient presented with bleeding from ear and impaired hearing with sign of head injury, there could be a fracture of
    A. Anterior cranial fossa
    B. Middle cranial fossa
    C. Posterior cranial fossa
    D. Mandibular fracture

48. A 15-Year-old otherwise healthy female patient presents at 1pm with a large, firm, brawny submandibular swelling on the right side. The patient has severe trismus, pyrexia and radiographs show a grossly carious lower right 6, the patient has some dysphagia but the tongue is not elevated, which of the following is/are indicated?
    A. Start antibiotics intramuscularly and drain the abscess under local anesthesia following admission a ward and medical care
    B. Start antibiotics intramuscularly and drain the abscess under general anesthesia following admission a ward and medical care
    C. Aspirate swelling and send to culture and sensitivity test to begin antibiotic therapy
    D. Give corticosteroids

49. A 29-year old patient taking 60mg hydrocortisone for the last one month, requires periodontal surgery
    A. It should not be carried out.
    B. The dose should be halved and then surgery carried out.

C. The dose should be doubled and then surgery performed

D. NO change in dose should be made and surgery should be carried out

50. Patient with iron deficiency anemia came for extraction of impacted wisdom tooth. Which of the following would be a contraindication for such a procedure?

A. HB = 7 mg/dl

B. HB = 11 mg/dl

C. HB = 12 mg/dl

D. HB = 13 mg/dl

51. Healthy pregnant woman came for extraction of lower wisdom tooth and she went into syncope. Which of the following is the most common cause?

A. Hypotension

B. Hypertension

C. High blood sugar

D. Low blood sugar

52. A 60-year-old patient suffered injuries to his lower half of face that suggested mandibular body fracture on examination. What is the most appropriate way of management of such a patient where there is no presence of teeth?

A. Gunning splint

B. Cap splint

C. Ribbon splint

D. All of the above

53. Long term effect of radiotherapy to oral mucosa is characterized by

A. Epithelium becomes more keratinized

B. Sub mucosa becomes highly vascular

C. Break down & delayed healing, submucosa less vascular

D. No sub mucosal fibrosis

54. Trauma to lower third of face is characterized by all of the following *except*
    - A. Fractures of the mandible are common at the angle of the mandible
    - B. Fractures of the mandible are affected by the muscle pull
    - C. Fractures of the mandible are usually characterized by sublingual hematoma
    - **D. CSF Rhinorrhea is a common finding**

55. A decision was made to treat a mandibular body fracture with closed reduction using ivy-eyelet wiring technique. Such a fracture mandible should be immobilized for an average of
    - A. 3 weeks
    - B. 6 weeks
    - C. 9 weeks
    - **D. 12 weeks**

56. In a worldwide consideration which part of the mandible can be considered to be suffering traumatic fractures the most?
    - A. Body
    - B. Angle
    - C. Symphysis
    - **D. Condyle**

57. A six-year-old child fell from a height and it was noticed on CT scan that one of the cortices of his mandible was fractured while other one was almost intact. What kind of fracture can be said to have occurred in him?
    - A. Displaced fracture
    - B. Telescopic fracture
    - **C. Greenstick fracture**
    - D. Overlapping fracture

58. An 8-year-old child fell on his chin while playing football and mid-symphysis fracture of lower jaw was noticed. What is the treatment of choice in such a patient?
    A. Intermaxillary fixation
    B. Cap splint with circumferential wiring
    C. Open reduction
    D. No treatment indicated

59. Submandibular gland is known to open in floor of the mouth by various openings but one of them forms a major duct to carry out secretions, which one of the following is that?
    A. Bartholin's duct
    B. Minor salivary gland's duct
    C. Stenson's duct
    D. Wharton's duct

60. Which of the following complication may result from injury to auriculotemporal nerve during removal of parotid tumor is
    A. Facial palsy
    B. Gustatory sweating
    C. Oro lingual paresthesia
    D. Anorexia

61. Duct for the parotid gland opens commonly in which region
    A. Upper 2nd molar
    B. Upper 3rd molar
    C. Lower 2nd molar
    D. Lower 3rd molar

62. Cross bar elevator which works on the wheel and axle principle has a mechanical advantage of
    A. 1.5 times the force applied
    B. 3 times the force applied
    C. 4.5 times the force applied
    D. 5.5 times the force applied

63. Which is the most preferred size of suture for skin sutures of face
    - A. 1/0
    - B. 2/0
    - C. 3/0
    - **D. 4/0**

64. Person with known history of diabetes mellitus has been on medications for past 10 years and needs a surgical extraction of 38. What is the best way of managing such a patient on the day of surgery?
    - A. Double the dose of Insulin
    - B. Double the quantity of breakfast
    - **C. Usual dose of insulin and Breakfast**
    - D. To not take insulin and come nil per oral

65. A 23-year-old male patient started having epileptic attack following overdose administration of local anesthesia and was not subsiding. The agent of choice to reverse status epilepticus induced by local anesthetic overdose is?
    - A. Phenobarbital
    - B. Epinephrine
    - C. Oxygen
    - **D. Diazepam**

66. A 40-year-old patient with severe maxillofacial injuries presented to the emergency in an unconscious state, he has to be
    - A. Immediately treated for maxillofacial injuries
    - B. Immediately Glasgow coma scale should be assessed
    - **C. Immediately airway should be secured**
    - D. Immediately examine for any associated fractures

67. A young female patient presented with a history of trauma to the face following a road traffic accident. On examination flattening of cheek on the left side was observed suggesting zygomatic arch fracture. The suggested radiograph will be
    - A. Occlusal view

B. Facial Profile Survey
C. Reverse - Towne Projection
D. Submentovertex Projection

68. A patient with continuity defect of mandible due to segmental resection of mandible is reconstructed using anterior iliac crest graft. This graft is an example for

A. Autogenous Corticocancellous bone graft
B. Autogenous Cancellous bone graft
C. Xenograft
D. Alloplastic bone graft

69. A 60-year-old patient with mandibular fracture was admitted post operatively in the ICU following open reduction and internal fixation. He suffered from nosocomial pneumonia. The most commonly involved organisms are

A. Gram positive organisms
B. Gram negative organisms
C. Mycoplasma
D. Virus infections

70. A female patient with a huge swelling on the face is diagnosed with buccal space infection. The method of treatment is

A. William's method of abscess drainage
B. Hilton's method of abscess drainage
C. Hilton's method of enucleation
D. William's method of decompression

71. A child was diagnosed with cleft of lip and palate upon birth, the initial step in management is

A. Nasoalveolar moulding
B. Surgery for cleft lip
C. Surgery for cleft palate
D. No treatment till adulthood

72. A patient with deep soft tissue laceration on the right mandibular region of the face associated with displaced parasymphysis of the right side walked into the emergency.
    A. The soft tissue is closed with layered sutures, and the patient is posted for fracture reduction the next day.
    B. The soft tissue debridement is done and stay sutures are placed. The patient is posted for fracture reduction the next day.
    C. The patient is posted for surgery immediately for both soft and hard tissue management.
    D. The patient is treated with closed reduction for parasymphysis fracture and stay sutures are placed for soft tissue.

73. A 50-year-old patient with history of chronic alcoholism requires multiple extractions. Which of the following conditions will he be more prone for?
    A. Increased PTT
    B. Increased blood sugar levels
    C. Decreased PTT
    D. Decreased INR

74. A 30-year-old patient had a severe cardiac arrest on the dental chair. After how much time of total oxygen obstruction to brain, permanent neurologic damage can occur?
    A. 1 min
    B. 2 mins
    C. 3 mins
    D. 4 mins

75. A patient with mild gnawing pain radiating around the right TMJ reported to our unit requesting extraction of upper and lower third molars of the right side. On examination, the muscles on the affected side were tender and the pain was radiating. Intraoral examination

revealed fully erupted, non-carious upper and lower third molars in occlusion. The most probable diagnosis is

A. MPDS
B. Pericoronitis
C. TMJ Dislocation
D. Periapical disease of lower third molar

76. A 25-year-old patient with upper canine impaction gave a radiographic picture of canine placed horizontally in the palate. How do we classify this position?

A. WHO Class I
B. WHO Class II
C. WHO Class III
D. WHO Class IV

77. A 30-year-old patient had a hard swelling on the palate in the midline measuring around0.5 cm to 1cm. The swelling was painless on palpation and non-mobile. What is the most probable diagnosis?

A. Lipoma
B. Torus palatinus
C. Fibroma
D. Osteosarcoma

78. A 40-year-old female patient presented with a swelling on the right side of the forehead since many years, and is gradually growing in size. On examination, it was well circumscribed, soft, and not attached to the underlining structure. Slip sign was positive. What is your diagnosis and management?

A. Sebaceous cyst, Aspiration of the contents
B. Infected follicle, Antibiotics
C. Lipoma, excision
D. Hyperplastic frontalis muscle shaving

79. An 18-year-old female patient was diagnosed with a radicular cyst extending from left canine to right canine of the mandible. The preferred treatment is
    A. Segmental resection of mandible
    B. Marsupialization
    C. Electrocautery
    D. Cryotherapy

80. A 60-year-old female patient, who was on long term bisphosphonate therapy for multiple myeloma, underwent extraction of 34 and 35. Postoperatively the mandibular bone was exposed and painful, with halitosis, swelling, and oro-cutaneous fistula. This condition is
    A. Dry socket
    B. Osteonecrosis
    C. Osteoradionecrosis
    D. Osteomyelitis

81. A 34-year-old patient presented with nasal bone fracture and deviated nasal septum with a history of trauma during boxing. It can be reduced using
    A. Ashleys and Walshams forceps
    B. Ashleys and Rowes disimpaction forceps
    C. Walshams and Rowes disimpaction forceps
    D. Index finger and thumb

82. A 40-year-old male patient with multiple facial fractures (PAN FACIAL TRAUMA) reported to the emergency unit with respiratory distress. The best way to secure airway is
    A. Blind nasal intubation
    B. Oral airway
    C. Emergency tracheostomy
    D. Mouth to mouth breathing

83. A 21-year-old female patient complained of large swelling on the right side of the face extending to neck, following the access opening of right lower second molar the previous day. Most likely she developed

    A. Abscess of submandibular space
    B. Cellulitis
    C. Chemical burn
    D. Allergic condition

84. A 25-year-old female patient presented with drooping of upper eyelid, drooling of saliva and inability to close the eye on the left side of the face following parotidectomy of the left side. The reason could be

    A. Injury to facial nerve
    B. Injury to trigeminal nerve
    C. Injury to parotid gland
    D. Injury to optic nerve

85. Following road traffic accident, a 50-year male patient presented with disturbed occlusion, ecchymosis in the greater palatine foramen region, ecchymosis in the buccal sulcus and mild mobility of the maxillary segment. And no tenderness over the nasal bridge or frontozygomatic suture region. The clinical diagnosis will be

    A. Dentoalveolar fracture
    B. Lefort I fracture
    C. Lefort II fracture
    D. Lefort III fracture

86. A 35-year-old female patient required extraction of left upper molars, but since she presented with exophthalmos, tremors and increased blood pressure the operating surgeon suspected

    A. Hypertension
    B. Hyperthyroidism
    C. Hypothyroidism
    D. Adrenal crisis

87. A 45-year-old male patient was ambulated to the emergency in a semiconscious state. He was diagnosed with mandibular, zygomatic and femoral fracture. Which of the fracture should be addressed first?
    A. Mandibular fracture
    B. Zygomatic fracture
    C. Femoral fracture
    D. Treatment should be postponed till he gains consciousness

88. A female with maxillofacial injuries was ambulated to the emergency following road traffic accident. She had feeble pulse, fall in blood pressure and tachycardia indicating hypovolemia. The circulatory volume should be immediately compensated with
    A. Blood of the same group
    B. Crystalloids
    C. Colloids
    D. Universal blood group

89. A patient with bilateral parasymphysis fracture of the mandible presenting with respiratory distress. The most likely cause will be
    A. Blood clot in the mouth
    B. Tongue falls back and obstructs the airway
    C. Soft palate obstructs the airway
    D. Hyoid bone is compressed

90. In a patient with bilateral parasymphysis fracture of the mandible presenting with respiratory distress the immediate measure taken to maintain airway is
    A. Pull the tongue with suture or towel clip
    B. Emergency tracheostomy
    C. Emergency cricothyroidectomy
    D. Jaw thrust method

91. While extracting a maxillary premolar the buccal root of the tooth got fractured, while trying to retrieve the root, it vanished from the socket. On radiograph the maxillary sinus was clear. Which is the next possible location for the root to escape
    A. Palatal space
    B. Buccal space
    C. Nasal cavity
    D. Orbital cavity

92. A young male patient was diagnosed with communited fracture of mandible. The ideal method of fixation is
    A. 2.5 mm plate
    B. 1.5 mm plate
    C. Dynamic compression plates with eccentric holes
    D. Reconstruction plates with central holes

93. A young female patient complained of painless swelling on the right side of the mandible which gradually increased in size. Histology revealed abnormal fibrous connective proliferation in which new non-maturing bone is seen, replacing the normal bone. The treatment is
    A. Enucleation of the lesion
    B. Bone shaving
    C. Mandibulectomy
    D. Radiation

94. A patient with suspected central giant cell granuloma was advised to check his levels of parathyroid hormone to rule out
    A. Primary hyperparathyroidism
    B. Primary hypoparathyroidism
    C. Primary hyperthyroidism
    D. Primary hypothyroidism

95. Which of the following is false?
    A. Gingival and palatal cyst of newborn is derived from dental lamina
    B. Epstein's pearl is found along the mid palatine suture
    C. Bohn's nodules are found along the mid palatine suture
    D. Palatal cyst of newborn persists into adult life

96. Which of the following glands is both endocrine and exocrine in nature?
    A. Pancreas
    B. Thyroid gland
    C. Sweat gland
    D. Pituitary gland

97. Which of the following GA agent is contraindicated in severe coronary artery disease
    A. Ketamine
    B. Fentanyl
    C. Thiopentanyl
    D. Xylocaine

98. Glenoid fossa is found in
    A. Orbital cavity
    B. Nasal cavity
    C. Middle cranial fossa
    D. **Temporal bone**

99. After you inject LA for maxillary 2nd molar, the patient's face becomes colorless with an extraoral swelling. Its due to
    A. Facial artery
    B. Plexus of vein
    C. Posterior alveolar nerve
    D. Maxillary artery

100. Patient reports to the clinic with the history multiple lesions of the head and neck manifested as nevi with is the most probable diagnosis?
    A. Peterson Kelly syndrome
    B. vander Woude syndrome
    C. Eagle syndrome
    D. Albright syndrome

101. All the following are examples of diseases causing aplastic anemia, *except*
    A. Hepatitis
    B. Pregnancy
    C. Cold hemoglobinuria
    D. PNH

102. A 5-year-old child came to the set up with an avulsed tooth. What is the most important factor that affects reimplantation of avulsed tooth
    A. Time since the avulsion
    B. Skill of dentist
    C. Contaminated roots
    D. Patient age

103. An increase in shear stress in a blood vessel results in which of the following changes?
    A. Decreased endothelin production
    B. Increased nitric oxide
    C. Increased rennin production
    D. Decreased prostacyclin production

104. Which of the following patterns is the characteristic of the response to nerve stimulation produced by a depolarizing neuromuscular agent
    A. A Lack of fade in response to train of four
    B. Increase in post-tetanic stimulation
    C. Tetanus is associated with fade in muscle response
    D. Fourth twitch of TOF disappears with 60-70% receptor occupancy

105. Drainage of tip of the tongue

   A. Sub lingual lymph nodes
   B. Submental lymph nodes
   C. Submandibular lymph nodes
   D. Parotid lymph nodes

106. Base of the flap should be wide for

   A. Healing
   B. For better suture placement
   C. Better blood supply to the wound.
   D. Nothing relevant

REFERENCES

Bagheri, S. C. (2014). *Clinical review of oral and maxillofacial surgery: A case-based approach.*

Balaji s. M. (2018). *Textbook of oral & maxillofacial surgery*. S.l.: Elsevier India.

Birn, H., & Winther, J. E. (1982). *Manual of minor oral surgery: A step by step atlas*. Copenhagen: Munksgaard.

Contemporary Oral and Maxillofacial Surgery. James R, Myron R, Edward Ellis. 6th Edition. Mosby; 2014.

Fonseca, R. J., Marciani, R. D., Turvey, T. A. (2009). *Oral andmaxillofacial surgery*. St. Louis, Mo: Saunders/Elsevier.

Hupp J. (2019). *Contemporary oral and maxillofacial surgery*. S.l.: Mosby.

Kruger, G. O. (1984). *Textbook of oral and maxillo-facial surgery*. Saint-Louis: Mosby.

Laskin, D. M. (2009). *Oral and maxillofacial surgery*. Delhi, India: A.I.T.B.S. Pub.

Malik, N. A. (2012). *Textbook of oral and maxillofacial surgery.*

Medical Emergencies in the Dental Office. Stanley Malamed. 7th Edition. Mosby. 2014.

Scully, C. (2014). *Scully; medical problems in dentistry.*

Textbook of Oral and Maxillofacial Surgery. B Srinivasan. 2nd Edn. Elsevier Science. 2015.

In: Scenario Based MCQ in Dentistry ISBN: 978-1-53617-298-0
Editors: M. Khursheed Alam et al.

Chapter 4

SCENARIO BASED MCQS IN PERIODONTOLOGY

Kiran Kumar Ganji, Ahmed Shawkat Hashem, Deepti Shrivastava and Ibrahim Alzoubi
Periodontics, College of Dentistry, Jouf University,
Aljouf, Saudi Arabia

This chapter describes scenario based MCQs dealing with field of Periodontology. Gingival and periodontal diseases, in their various forms have afflicted humans since the dawn of history, and studies in paleopathology have indicated that destructive periodontal disease as evidenced by bone loss affected early humans in such diverse cultures as ancient Egypt and early pre-Columbian America. The earliest historical records dealing with medical topics reveal an awareness of periodontal disease and the need for the treatment. Periodontal diseases are considered to be complex diseases of multi-factorial origin and variable treatment outcomes. While the periodontal diseases are unquestionably initiated by bacteria, it is the individual's host inflammatory response and other superimposed modifying and predisposing factors that ultimately determine the clinical presentation and outcome of the many and varied forms of periodontal disease. Specifically, disease progression appears to be regulated by environmental and genetic factors specific to the individual. Thus, the practice of contemporary periodontics dictates that the unique inflammatory response and associated controlling factors must be taken into account when diagnosing, treating, and managing the periodontal diseases. The goals of traditional periodontal therapy have been to eliminate deep pockets, eliminate gingival bleeding, and achieve meticulous plaque control in all patients. Accordingly, periodontal treatment has become more focused and now aims to reduce all undesirable clinical findings to as low a level as is possible, practically, biologically, and individually. In general, this is achieved by: (i) treating the periodontal diseases as opportunistic infections modified by host inflammatory responses, (ii) controlling the inflammation and infection, (iii) reducing predisposing factors, (iv) controlling modifying factors, and (v) providing continuous assessment and supportive periodontal care.

1. Patient reported with chief complaint of bleeding gums in lower posterior region. Clinical examination shows deep pocket of 7 mm distal to 36 While other areas show shallow pockets with clinical attachment loss in the range of 2-3 mm. Diagnosis was made as chronic periodontitis with trauma from occlusion in relation to 36.Which group of PDL fibers could become affected in the region of 36?
   A. Oblique group
   B. Alveolar crest group
   C Transseptal group
   D. Horizontal group

2. A 60 years male patient reported with chief complaint of bleeding gums. Clinical examination shows generalized bleeding on probing without attachment loss. What could be the reason for not developing periodontitis in this case?
   A. Presence of only gram positive bacteria in the plaque
   B. Good host resistance

C. Absence of systemic disease
D. Presence of all teeth.

3. A 57 years male patient reported with chief complaint of bleeding gum and bad breath. Clinical examination shows generalized deep pockets with clinical attachment loss in the range of 5-6 mm. Radiograph shows generalized horizontal bone loss. What could be the reason for developing periodontitis in this patient?
   A. Due to old age
   B. Due to loss of few teeth
   C. Occurrence of periodontopathic bacteria in plaque
   D. Due to generalized attrition of teeth.

4. 35 years female patient reported with complaint of pain in gingiva and burning during urination, clinical examination shows a patchy distribution of bright red areas involving marginal and attached gingiva, in addition there was Conjunctivitis. What would be your diagnosis?
   A. Lichen planus
   B. Mucous membrane pemphigoid
   C. Pemphigus
   D. ANUG

5. 23 years female patient reported with complaint of redness of gingiva without pain, clinical examination shows diffused erythema of marginal, interdental and attached gingiva. What would be your diagnosis?
   A. Moderate form of desquamative gingivitis
   B. Mild form of desquamative gingivitis
   C. Acute herpetic gingivostomatitis
   D. Acute streptococcal gingivitis

6. Patient came with complaint of bad breath; clinical examination shows generalized deep periodontal pockets. What substance produced in periodontal pockets that is responsible for bad breath?
   A. B-Glucoroniodase
   B. Collaginase
   C. Aspertate amino transferase
   D. Hydrogen sulphide

7. Patient came with complaint of bad breath, clinical examination shows healthy gingiva, no periodontal pockets, no loss of attachment. What could be the possible cause for bad breath?
   A. Poor oral hygiene
   B. Lung abscess
   C. Deposits on tongue
   D. Healing extraction socket

8. 12-year male patient reported with mental deficiency and growth retardation and severe destruction of periodontium.
   A. Down syndrome
   B. Papillonlefevre syndrome
   C. Candidiasis
   D. ANUG

9. Gingiva appears red, friable and located in the oral aspect of attached gingiva and sometimes it may be associated with rapidly progressive periodontitis are the feature of
   A. Sarcoidosis
   B. Plasma cell gingivitis
   C. Peripheral giant cell granuloma
   D. Pyogenic granuloma

10. A female patient presents with swelling in lower anterior region. Histopathology examination reveals prominent endothelial

proliferation with capillary formation and associated inflammation is the feature of

A. Central giant cell granuloma
B. Pregnancy tumor
C. Plasma cell granuloma
D. Peripheral giant cell granuloma

11. Patient came with complaint of esthetic problem in lower anterior region after commencement of treatment for ANUG. Clinical examination shows presence of defects in gingival contour at interdental area in lower anterior region. Such gingival defects are called

A. Stillman's clefts
B. McCall's festoon
C. Reverse architecture
D. Gingival craters

12. A 49 years male patient with periodontal disease gave a history of excessive thirst and hunger from past 5 years. In addition, he also gave the history of eye surgery one year back. One of the following is the medical emergency related with above mentioned condition

A. Diabetes
B. Hypertension
C. Hemophilia
D. Hepatitis

13. A 42 years male patient with chronic periodontitis was undertaken for the regenerative surgery. During the procedure, patient experienced pain in chest which was associated with stress. One of the following is the medical emergency related with above mentioned condition

A. Hepatitis
B. Leukemia
C. Myocardial infarction
D. Angina

14. Patient came with complain of bleeding gums in lower anterior region. Clinical examination shows presence of both supra and sub gingival plaque. Which one of the following bacteria may not be the cause of bleeding gums?
    A. Streptococci Mutans
    B. P. Gingivalis
    C. Treponema Denticola
    D. Taneralla Forsythia

15. Patient complains of bad breath, Clinical examination shows deep periodontal pocket 5-7 mm in the region of maxillary and mandibular right and left first molar and central incisor, Name the type of plaque responsible for such region
    A. Attached Sub Gingival Plaque
    B. Unattached Sub Gingival Plaque
    C. Marginal Plaque
    D. Attachment Plaque

16. Patient reported with complaint of bleeding gums. Clinical examination shows presence of generalized subgingival calculus. Which type of plaque is responsible for such type of calculus?
    A. Supragingival plaque
    B. Subgingival unattached plaque
    C. Subgingival attached plaque
    D. Marginal plaque

17. Patient came with complaint of bleeding gums. Clinical examination shows continuous bands of heavy calculus on lingual side of 31,32,33,41,42,43 areas with clinical attachment loss in the range of 5-7mm without tooth mobility. What could be the reason for not having mobility 31,32,33,41,42,43?
    A. Minimal attachment loss
    B. Minimal bone loss
    C. Minimal loss of supporting tissue
    D. Artificially holding the tooth by big chunk of calculus

18. An 18 year old boy complains of tooth pain after bitng on an olive pit. The cause for this pain of 1 day duration is
    - **A. Acute trauma**
    - B. Occlusal disharmony
    - C. Secondary trauma
    - D. Primary trauma

19. A 25-year-old male complains of mobility in his lower molars after a prosthetic replacement of his upper molars 15 days back. On examination there is no clinical attachment loss or pocket formation in the teeth and the oral hygiene is good. The reason for this mobility
    - A. Acute trauma
    - B. Occlusal disharmony
    - **C. Secondary trauma**
    - D. Primary trauma

20. A 20-year-old patient came with a chief complaint of severe pain in relation to the mandibular right second premolar. On examination there was a small abscess in the attached gingiva and a lobster shell was found embedded. The likely diagnosis is
    - A. Periodontal pockets
    - **B. Acute gingival abscess**
    - C. Periodontal abscess
    - D. Periapical abscess

21. A 35-year-old male patient comes with a chief complaint of food impaction in relation to lower left molar. On examination a pocket 6mm in depth is found. The following measurement will help to determine, clinically, the architecture of the underlying bone
    - A. Probing pocket depth .
    - **B. Clinical Attachment loss**
    - C. Width of attached gingiva
    - D. Width of keratinized gingiva

22. Examination of a 35-year-old male patient attending the outpatient clinic of the department of Periodontics reveals enlargement of the right submandibular lymph node. All of the following periodontal conditions may result in enlarged lymph nodes *except*
    A. Primary herpetic gingivostomatitis
    B. Necrotizing ulcerative gingivitis (NUG)
    C. Acute periodontal abscess
    D. Gingivitis

23. Patient came with complaint of bleeding gums in lower anterior region. Clinical examination shows 5-6 mm pocket. 31 tooth on labial surface has CAL 5 mm. What will be the distance between CEJ to the crest of marginal bone?
    A. 5 mm
    B. 3 mm
    C. 7 mm
    D. 8 mm

24. Patient came with complaint of dull pain in lower right region. Clinical examination shows deep pocket distal of 45 with blunting of interdental papilla and loss of proximal contact between 45,46. Radiograph shows angular bone loss. Which part of alveolar bone must have been affected?
    A. Cortical bone
    B. Compact bone
    C. Alveolar bone proper
    D. Buccal plate

25. Patient came for the replacement of missing 26 tooth by implant bearing prosthesis. Clinical examination shows vertical ridge defect. Name the type of bone blocks useful for vertical ridge augmentation.
    A. Autogenous bone block from symphysis region
    B. Autogenous bone block from ramus region
    C. Autogenous bone block from iliac crest
    D. DFDBA bone block

26. Patient came for routine dental checkup. Clinical examination shows healthy gingiva without periodontal pockets. Radiographic examination shows hypercementosis of entire dentition. What could be the possible cause?
    A. Scleroderma
    B. Fibrous dysplasia
    C. Paget's disease
    D. Osteopetrosis

27. Patient came with complaint of pain in lower front region while taking cold water. Clinical examination shows healthy gingiva without caries, abrasion or erosion in lower anterior region. There was slight gingival recession on labial surface of 31,32,41,42. What could be the cause?
    A. Faulty brushing technique
    B. Use of tooth powder for cleaning of teeth
    C. Exposure of dentin due to gap junction between Cementum and enamel
    D. Use of worn out toothbrush

28. Patient came with the complaint of bleeding gums. Clinical diagnosis was established as chronic gingivitis. The primary cause may be
    A. Plaque
    B. Calculus
    C. Food Debris
    D. Materia Alba

29. A patient with a known case of localized aggressive periodontitis was given 100 mg antibiotic for first day twice daily and later on once daily for 14 days. This drug is
    A. Minocycline
    B. Penicillin
    C. Metronidazole
    D. Doxycycline

30. A 32 years male patient having a history of aggressive periodontitis was found to be refractory to tetracycline therapy and so he was advised another antibiotic
    - A. Azithromycin
    - B. Clindamycin
    - **C. Ciprofloxacin**
    - D. Tetracycline

31. A 26 years old female patient came for a dental checkup and on examination she was found to be a case of generalized aggressive periodontitis. Combination antibiotic therapy was given as an adjunct to scaling and root planning. Combination drug therapy can be
    - **A. Metronidazole plus amoxicillin**
    - B. Amoxicillin plus tetracycline
    - C. Amoxicillin plus Ciprofloxacin
    - D. Clindamycin plus metronidazole

32. A male patient was indicated for definite curettage procedure. ENAP is definitive sub-gingival curettage to be performed by
    - A. Blade
    - **B. Knife**
    - C. Both blade and knife
    - D. Curette

33. A student was performing gingival curettage. Among all instruments, which one of the following instruments is not used during gingival curettage procedure?
    - A. Scissors
    - B. Curettes
    - **C. Surgical Blade**
    - D. Lasers

34. For elimination of suprabony pocket regardless of their depth, if pocket wall is fibrous and firm, gingivectomy is indicated when
    A. Need for bone surgery
    B. The bottom of pocket located apical to MGJ
    C. Aesthetic consideration particularly in anterior maxilla
    D. the bottom of pocket located coronal to mucogingival junction

35. A 25-year-old boy reports with a single-root stump present in the maxillary anterior region and wants to replace it with a fixed prosthesis. The quality of bone in the area is very good with adequate width and length available. He wants the tooth to be replaced immediately since his esthetics is compromised. The treatment of choice would be
    A. One-stage implants
    B. Two-stage implants
    C. Delayed implants
    D. Immediate implants

36. The percentage of bone to implant contact of roughened surface implants range from
    A. 10-20
    B. 21-30
    C. 31-40
    D. < = 41

37. With respect regenerative periodontal therapy, it was decided to use Enamel matrix derivative (Emdogain®) over other regenerative materials. Emdogain promotes osteoblastic proliferation as it is composed mainly of
    A. amelin
    B. enamelins
    C. amelogenin
    D. enamel tuftelin

38. What is a good predictor of the onset of necrotizing ulcerative periodontitis in HIV-infected patients?
    - A. Candida infection
    - B. Survival less than 6 months
    - C. CD8+ cell counts < 500 cells/mm^3
    - **D. CD4+ cell counts < 200 cells/mm^3**

39. The application of controlled lateral forces on dental implants produces
    - **A. increases in bone density**
    - B. reductions in bone density
    - C. increases in bone to implant contact
    - D. reductions in bone to implant contact

40. In which epithelial cell layer does proliferation of gingival keratinocytes primarily occur?
    - **A. Stratum basale**
    - B. Stratum corneum
    - C. Stratum spinosum
    - D. Stratum granulosum

41. Which of the following small proteins is found only in bone where it is secreted by osteoblasts and binds to the bone minerals?
    - A. Fibronectin
    - **B. Osteocalcin**
    - C. Osteonectin
    - D. Tenascin

42. Osteoprotegerin ligand (OPG-L or RANK-L) is a bone-resorbing factor released by T cells and
    - **A. osteoblasts**
    - B. neutrophils
    - C. osteoclasts
    - D. B-lymphocytes

43. Which of the following microorganisms has been associated with linear gingival erythema?
    A. C. albicans
    B. C. rectus
    C. H. capsulatum
    D. H. aphrophilus

44. A gingival reaction that has been attributed to pyrophosphates in tartar control toothpastes is
    A. sloughing
    B. pigmentation
    C. spontaneous bleeding
    D. papillary enlargement

45. What is the mechanism of action for topically applied chlorhexidine gluconate?
    A. Inhibits cell wall synthesis
    B. Disrupts membrane permeability
    C. Interferes with DNA replication
    D. Inactivates bacterial protein sulfhydryl groups

46. The initial thickening of the gingival tissues following root coverage using a bioresorbable membrane gradually decreases over several months and is thought to parallel
    A. scar formation
    B. reduction in edema
    C. resorption of adjacent alveolar bone
    D. maturation of the granulation tissue

47. The mechanism of povidone-iodine includes oxidation of all of the following *except*
    A. nucleotides
    B. lipopolysaccharide
    C. thiol moieties of amino acids
    D. hydroxy moieties of amino acids

48. During the progression of destructive periodontitis, which of the gingival fiber groups usually remains and can be easily visualized in mesio-distal histological sections?
    A. Circular
    B. Transseptal
    C. Dentogingival
    D. Alveologingival

49. All of the following function primarily as opsonins *except*
    A. IgG
    B. C3b
    C. IgE
    D. IgM

50. Which of the following is elevated in serum for both periodontitis and cardiovascular disease?
    A. IL-4
    B. CRP
    C. IL-3
    D. TGF-β

51. Which of the following disease entities may result in a total lack of cementum formation in the primary anterior teeth?
    A. Niemann-Pick
    B. Letterer-Siwe
    C. Hypophosphatasia
    D. Ectodermal dysplasia

52. Diabetic patient presented to the clinic complaining of gingival inflammation and bleeding, which factor matters most?
    A. Regular brushing
    B. Efficient scaling and curettage
    C. Antimicrobial therapy
    D. Control of diabetic condition

53. Radiographic examination of a patient revealed mirror image arc-shaped resorption affecting right and left lower first molars, and upper left central incisor. The most probable diagnosis of this patient would be
    A. Localized Chronic Periodontitis
    B. Localized Aggressive Periodontitis
    C. Generalized Aggressive Periodontitis
    D. Generalized Chronic Periodontitis

54. Periodontitis patient under anticoagulant therapy using Warfarin should not be treated with the following antibiotic as it interacts with Warfarin?
    A. Amoxicillin
    B. Metronidazole
    C. Ciprofloxacin
    D. Tavanic

55. Patient presented to the clinic for screening complaining of excessive salivation, this is more common in
    A. Chronic periodontitis
    B. Aggressive Periodontitis
    C. Necrotizing ulcerative gingivitis
    D. Periodontal abscess

56. Apically positioned flap is contraindicated in case of
    A. 1-wall bony defect management
    B. 2-wall bony defect management
    C. 3-wall bony defect management
    D. Class III furcation defect management

57. Contraindications of root resection include
    A. Horizontal bone loss
    B. Vertical bone loss
    C. Gingival inflammation
    D. Age of the patient

58. Patient with periodontal disease was treated in the clinic, after scaling and root planing, healing occur by
    A. Connective tissue attachment
    B. Long junctional epithelium
    C. New bone formation
    D. New attached periodontal ligament fibers

59. The periodontal tissues comprise which of the following tissues
    A. Gingiva and the PDL
    B. Gingiva, PDL, and alveolar bone
    C. Gingiva, PDL, alveolar bone, and cementum
    D. Gingiva, PDL, alveolar bone, cementum, and enamel

60. A student came to the clinic with severe pain, foul taste, and highly inflamed interdental papilla, most probable diagnosis is
    A. Gingivitis
    B. ANUG
    C. Periodontitis
    D. Gingival enlargement

61. Patient came to the clinic and his medical history revealed chronic renal failure, the patient undergo dialysis. Periodontal treatment should be done
    A. The day before dialysis
    B. On the day of dialysis
    C. One day after dialysis
    D. One week after dialysis

62. Patient came to the clinic complaining of inflamed gingiva, loss of gingival contour, and recession. The best tooth brushing technique to be prescribed
    A. Modified Bass
    B. Modified Stillman
    C. Charter
    D. Scrub

63. When performing crown lengthening, we should not violate the Biologic width which measures
    A. 1 mm
    B. 2 mm
    C. 3 mm
    D. 4 mm

64. We should treat ANUG until the disease completely disappears. Otherwise, it will change to generalized Chronic Periodontitis.
    A. Both sentences are true
    B. Both sentences are false
    C. 1st true, 2nd false
    D. 1st false, 2nd true

65. Patient came with severe pain related to right 1st mandibular molar, there's no swelling related, pulp test is negative, no evidence in radiograph. Diagnosis is
    A. Irreversible pulpitis
    B. Suppurative periodontal abscess
    C. Periapical abscess
    D. Acute periodontal abscess

66. Purpose of subgingival scaling is
    A. To remove calculus
    B. To remove necrotic cementum
    C. To make root surface biocompatible
    D. To remove gingival lining

67. Upon radiographic and clinical evaluation of a patient with periodontal destruction, severe bone loss was detected despite very slight calculus deposits, which is a characteristic picture for
    A. Necrotizing ulcerative periodontitis
    B. Generalized Chronic periodontitis
    C. Generalized aggressive periodontitis
    D. Refractory periodontitis

68. Differences between acute necrotizing ulcerative gingivitis (ANUG) and acute herpetic gingivostomatitis (AHGS) are
    A. ANUG occur in dental papilla while AHGS appear as diffuse erythematous gingiva
    B. ANUG occur in young adult while AHGS occur in children
    C. ANUG can cause necrosis while AHGS can cause multiple ulcers
    D. All of the above

69. A 47 years old patient came to the clinic suffering from dull pain in the upper right posterior teeth. Periodontal examination revealed presence of pockets in between upper first and second molars with clinical attachment loss ranging from 3 to 4 mm. The most probable diagnosis is
    A. Localized moderate chronic periodontitis
    B. Generalized moderate chronic periodontitis
    C. Generalized mild to moderate chronic periodontitis
    D. Localized mild to moderate chronic periodontitis

70. Patient having overhanging restoration should be managed by its removal because
    A. It tears the gingival fibers
    B. It stimulates inflammatory reaction directly
    C. Its removal permits more effective plaque control
    D. It leads to open contact area

71. A patient presented to the dental clinic with gingival recession, extending to the mucogingival junction with slight periodontal loss in the interdental area. The patient is complaining of esthetic appearance. What is the diagnosis of this case?
    A. Class I gingival recession
    B. Class II gingival recession
    C. Class III gingival recession
    D. Class IV gingival recession

72. A 58 years old male presents with gingival enlargement in the upper anterior region and gives a positive history of hypertensive medication. The enlargement involves papilla and the marginal gingiva. The enlargement disappears after oral prophylaxis. What is classification for this gingival enlargement?
    A. Drug induced overgrowth
    B. Inflammatory gingival enlargement
    C. Enlargements due to systemic diseases or conditions
    D. False enlargement

73. A patient complains of generalized enlargement of gingiva. On examination petechiae, ecchymosis and spontaneous bleeding was seen. On histopathologic examination gingiva was infiltrated with premature WBCs. Bone marrow examination showed inhibition of normal stem cells function. What is the most probable etiology?
    A. Vitamin C deficiency
    B. **Leukemic gingiva**
    C. Cyclosporine induced gingival overgrowth
    D. Pyogenic granuloma

74. A 26-year-old female having gingival inflammation that involves the papillary, marginal and attached gingiva of about 2 or 3 teeth in a full dentition. What would be your diagnosis?
    A. localized marginal gingivitis
    B. generalized marginal gingivitis
    C. **localized diffuse gingivitis**
    D. Generalized diffuse gingivitis

75. Dentist is scaling on 16 (right upper 1st molar) and taking a finger rest on 44 (right lower 1st premolar). This type of finger rest is called as
    A. Conventional
    B. Cross arch
    C. Opposite arch
    D. Finger on finger

76. A female patient of 45 years of age was diagnosed as chronic generalized marginal gingivitis with localized periodontitis irt 14,15,16,25,26 and 27. She had pocket depth of 6mm in relation to these teeth for which she has underwent periodontal flap surgery. On recall visit after 3 months the probing depth has reduced to 3mm irt, 25,26,27 whereas it is 4mm irt to 14,15,16. What would be your treatment planning during recall visit?
    A. Full mouth scaling and polishing
    B. Full mouth Scaling and root planning irt 14,15,16
    C. Full mouth Scaling and gingival curettage irt 14,15,16
    D. Periodontal flap surgery irt 14,15,16

77. A Male patient 56 years of age has Class II Gingival recession (W. D. Miller) in relation to 42and 43. The best treatment option given during preventive phase will be
    A. Scaling and Root planning
    B. Scaling and gingival curettage
    C. Root planning alone
    D. Free gingival graft

78. Tooth no 24 is indicated for crown lengthening. On examination, the attached gingiva is < 3mm. Which technique can be used to perform crown lengthening?
    A. Gingivectomy
    B. Apically displaced flap without bone recontouring
    C. Apically displaced flap with bone recontouring
    D. papilla preservation flap with bone recontouring

79. A patient presented to the dental clinic with supragingival calculus & inflammation of the gingiva in relation to 42,41,31,32 with 4 mm pocket & 2mm of apparent recession in the same region. The diagnosis would be
    A. Localized moderate chronic periodontitis
    B. Localized mild chronic periodontitis

C. Localized severe chronic periodontitis
D. Generalized severe chronic periodontitis

80. A female patient having gnawing pain and itching sensation irt tooth no # 36. On examination the depth of penetration of probe from base of the sulcus/pocket to gingival margin was 6 mm. On radiographic examination there is vertical bone resorption. It depicts
    A. Infrabony pocket
    B. Normal healthy gingiva
    C. Suprabony pocket
    D. Gingival pocket

81. A 20-year girl came with the following sign and symptoms: The area distal to 37 is Red, swollen, suppurating and painful. Patient has difficulty in opening of the mouth, foul taste and there is swelling of the cheek in the region of the angle of the jaw and lymphadenitis. Give the diagnosis of the condition
    A. Acute necrotizing ulcerative gingivitis
    B. Acute Pericoronitis
    C. Acute herpectic gingivostomatitis
    D. Malignant melanoma

82. A 30-year-old boy came gives a history of Localized, painful, rapidly expanding lesions in marginal gingival irt 23 which becomes fluctuant & pointed with surface orifice within 24-48 hours. What could be your diagnosis?
    A. Chronic inflammatory enlargement
    B. Acute inflammatory enlargement
    C. Sarcoidosis
    D. Plasma cell gingivitis

83. A male patient 48 years of age on examination it was found that, Tooth no #36 has 6mm pocket depth and is indicative of hemisection, which flap technique will be performed?

A. Modified Widman flap
B. Distal molar surgery
C. Papilla preservation flap
D. All of the above

84. Tooth no #24 is indicated for crown lengthening. It has fenestration on the buccal aspect with narrow band of attached gingiva, which flap technique is indicated?
    A. Modified Widman flap
    B. Partial thickness apically positioned flap
    C. Full thickness apically positioned flap
    D. Modified flap operation

85. A female patient 45 years of age, visited our dental clinic with itching sensation irt 26. On clinical and radiological examination, a pockets depth of 6 mm was found along with Grade II furcation involvement respectively. Which flap technique will be ideal for this case?
    A. Modified Widman operation
    B. Papilla preservation flap
    C. Apically positioned flap
    D. Modified flap operation

86. A male patient on 36 has been given a crown one month back. He developed pain and swelling in that region. On examination, it was found there is redness and swelling with bleeding on probing in that region. On bone sounding biologic width is found less than 2mm what could be the possible reason?
    A. Inadequate oral hygiene
    B. Violation of biologic width
    C. supragingival placement of the crown
    D. food impaction

87. A 54-year-old male patient intraoperatively found to have ledge in relation to 26,27 areas what would be the treatment options?

A. Regenerative techniques by using bone grafts
B. Regenerative techniques by using resorbable membrane alone
C. Resective osseous surgery
D. Gingivectomy

88. A male patient 45 years of age presents with recession (Class II) defect with 11,12,21. On examination there is sufficient width of attached gingiva and patient does not want a second surgical site. Which of the following procedures is most suitable for treating this patient?
A. Connective tissue graft
B. Coronally displaced Flap
C. Free gingival graft
D. Double papilla flap

89. A 5-year-old female child presents with dry scaly skin mainly in the hand and leg extremities. The patient gives history of reddened and swollen gingiva. During the 1st year after eruption of deciduous teeth it was followed by rapid destruction of periodontium manifested by noticeable, extensive resorption of bone and deep periodontal pockets with exudates in response to the slightest pressure. What could be the probable diagnosis?
A. Down syndrome
B. Papillon lefevre syndrome
C. cyclic neutropenia
D. lazy leukocyte syndrome

90. Tooth no #42 has 3 mm of Class II gingival recession (P. D. Miller) in the labial aspect. Tension test is positive with mandibular labial frenum. What would be the treatment sequence? 1) Frenectomy, 2) Scaling and polishing, 3) Free gingival graft, 4) Root planning.
A. 3,4,2,1
B. 2,3,4,1
C. 2,4,1,3
D. 1,3,2,4

91. Patient suffers from gingivitis with enlarged, hemorrhagic bluish, red gingiva, and hemorrhage in the periodontal ligament. He is diagnosed as suffering from Scurvy. Which component of the food need to be introduced?

    A. Vitamin B
    B. Vitamin D
    C. Vitamin C
    D. Vitamin A

92. A 49 years old male patient comes with a chief complain of bleeding gums in upper left back side of the teeth. On examination there is whitish yellow colour deposit which is not removed by water jet. Intra-operatively this deposit is easy to remove from scaler. What it could be?

    A. Material alba
    B. Supragingival calculus
    C. Intrinsic stains
    D. Serumal calculus

93. A 56 old male patient presents with following sign in the oral cavity.

    1. Gingival poly with 35
    2. Pocket formation and bone loss with 46,47,48
    3. Mucosal drying and chelosis

    Which systemic condition he might be suffering from?

    A. Hypertension
    B. Diabetes
    C. Hyperthyroidism
    D. COPD

94. A 39 years old female patient reported to the dental clinic with the following sign and symptoms i.e., ulceration of the oral mucosa and oro pharynx, dysphagia, glossitis and weakness. Which condition the patient might be suffering from?

    A. Aplastic anemia

B. Thrombocytopenia
C. Plummer Vinson syndrome
D. Chediak Higashi syndrome

95. A 40 years old male patient working in a chemical industry and does not have history of taking tobacco in any form. On examination his teeth are showing blue green stains. Which component would be responsible for this stain?
A. Tea/Coffee
B. Mercury
C. *Flavobacterium lutescens*
D. Tetracycline

96. A 52-year-old male patient, intraoperatively presents with ledges in the 16 & 17 region, which LASER can be used to treat the defect?
A. CO_2
B. Er: YAG
C. Argon
D. Diode

97. In a 54-year-old male patient there is calculus deposition seen in mandibularlingual anteriors and maxillary posteriors. Which theory of calculus formation is most appropriate in this case?
A. Transformation theory
B. CO_2 Theory
C. Enzymatic theory
D. Bacterial theory

98. In a 55-year-old male patient there is a linear steel grey gingival pigmentation associated with localized inflammation. It is because of
A. Bismuth intoxication
B. Mercury intoxication
C. Lead intoxication
D. Arsenic intoxication

99. A 17-year-old girl girl present with clinical attachment loss in relation to incisors and molars and inconsistent amount of plaque with the amount of periodontal destruction. What type of bone loss is expected in the present scenario?
    A. Horizontal bone loss
    B. Generalized bone loss
    C. Vertical loss of alveolar bone around 1st molars &incisors
    D. horizontal loss of alveolar bone around 1st molars & incisors

100. A post graduate student wants to detect Aa, Pg and Pi chair side for research purpose based on ELISA method of detection, which kit can be used?
    A. Perioscan
    B. Evalusite
    C. Omnigene
    D. Periotron

REFERENCES

Chapple, Iain LC. *Periodontal Medicine - A Window on the Body*. Quintessence Publishing Company., 2006. ISBN: 9781850970798.

Lindhe, *J. Clinical Periodontology & Implant Dentistry*. Blackwell., 2004. 978-1405160995.

Nuemann, Takei GR. Carranza. *Clinical Peridontology*, Vol 2, 2012. Saunders. ISBN: 9781437704168.

Reddy, Shantipriya. Essentials of Clinical Periodontology and Periodontics. *eepya J.*, 2011. ISBN: 9789350250372.

Serge, Dibart; Mamdouh Karima. Dibert, S. *Practical Periodontal Plastic Surgery*. Wiley-Blackwell, 2006. ISBN: 978-0813822686.

In: Scenario Based MCQ in Dentistry ISBN: 978-1-53617-298-0
Editors: M. Khursheed Alam et al.

Chapter 5

SCENARIO-BASED MCQS IN CONSERVATIVE DENTISTRY

Azhar Iqbal, Fayyaz Alam and Magda Eleraky, PhD
Conservative Dentistry, Department of Conservative Dentistry and Endodontics, College of Dentistry, Jouf University, Aljouf, Saudi Arabia

Conservative dentistry is the backbone of dentistry with equal emphasis on preventive and restorative treatments. A graduate is initiated into this world by introducing the mysteries behind enamel, dentin, cementum and pulp organ. The discussion then gradually moves to the microbiology, histopathology and epidemiology of caries. Caries risk assessment and role of diet and diet counselling are discussed threadbare. Ever since WHO declared the world-wide campaign on dental caries, focus has been on prevention of dental caries. Role of fluorides and efficacy of fluoridation in bringing down the DMF index is now well acknowledged. Diagnosis of incipient caries and early intervention are given lots of importance in the modern era.

Introduction of adhesive restorative materials and pit and fissure sealants have almost pushed back conventional methods of tooth preparation and lay focus on minimally invasive techniques. Multiple facets of adhesive restorations like tooth preparation, etching, bonding is discussed along with the guidelines on aesthetic restorations. However, a student of dentistry cannot altogether ignore G V Black's concepts of cavity preparation. Topics have been included to help the graduate revise the 'extension for prevention' concept and amalgam restoration. Complex amalgam restoration and management of wear lesions are also given due importance. Extra care has been taken to discuss contentious topics like galvanism, hypersensitivity, microleakage and amalgam toxicity. A short discourse on vital pulp therapeutic procedures like direct and indirect pulp capping have also been added so as to complete the overview on operative dentistry.

1. On a bitewing radiograph, a carious lesion is visible on the approximal surface of the upper molar. The tooth needs to be restored if
    A. the caries has involved the enamel
    B. the carious lesion is cavitated and involves the deeper dentin
    C. the caries has not changed in size since a previous radiograph was taken
    D. the carious lesion involves the root surface

2. Quantitative laser fluorescence uses incident blue light to illuminate the tooth. The healthy tooth enamel fluoresces a green colour, which is captured by the intra-oral camera, while the blue light is filtered out. Quantitative laser fluorescence allows the detection of carious lesions
    A. which are seen as dark areas over the affected enamel
    B. because of the decreased scattering of incident light
    C. which are seen as red areas over the affected enamel
    D. but cannot be used to monitor the enamel remineralisation following regular application of fluoride varnish

3. In carious root surface lesions that have arrested, they usually
   - A. appear soft when probed
   - **B. appear brown in colour and feel hard when probed**
   - C. have heavily infected dentine
   - D. lie close to or beneath the gingival margin

4. The minimum width of an occlusal cavity preparation is limited by the minimum width that can be used in the manufacture of diamond and tungsten carbide burs. The ideal minimum width of a cavity outline is therefore
   - A. between 0.5 and 0.8 mm
   - B. between 1 and 1.2 mm
   - **C. between 0.8 and 1 mm**
   - D. between 1.4 and 1.5 mm

5. What is the average life-span of an extensive amalgam restoration placed by an experienced dentist?
   - A. 5–8 years
   - **B. 10–15 years**
   - C. 16–20 years
   - D. Over 20 years

6. A 45 year old male patient came to you in the Operative clinic with the complaint of sensitivity. On Clinical examination it has been found that he is having abfraction lesion in the cervical areas of upper and lower molar and premolar region. These abfraction lesions
   - A. are caused by toothbrush abrasion
   - B. are shallow, bowl-shaped cervical lesions that affect the molar teeth
   - **C. result from the propagation of cracks through the cervical enamel**
   - D. occur at the sites of wear on the occlusal surface

7. You placed an amalgam restoration in maxillary right first molar. Immediately after the placement the amalgam restoration is carved so that
   A. centric occlusion is coincident with centric relation
   B. the teeth meet evenly in centric occlusion
   C. B the teeth meet evenly in centric relation
   D. D the amalgam avoids any contact with the opposing tooth

8. In the Operative clinic you have decided to place a complex amalgam restoration in tooth no 36 by using dentinal pins as an additional method of retention. Regarding Dentinal pins which of the following option is correct
   A. Pins should be placed in dentine at about 1 mm from the enamel-dentine junction
   B. Pins should rarely be placed parallel to the external root surface
   C. Pins should engage dentine to a depth of 3–4 mm
   D. Pins cannot be adjusted after placement, as this will cause their fracture

9. A young 25 years old patient came to you with ahx of dull pain and sensitivity. On clinical and radiographic examination you have found that he is having a proximal carious lesion with sound and intact marginal ridge in tooth no 46. You decided to place the glass ionomer restoration by using tunnel technique. This treatment
   A. provides good resistance to further demineralisation
   B. is improved with prior etching of the enamel and dentine with phosphoric acid before restoration placement
   C. allows effective caries removal
   D. results in a reduced strength for the marginal ridge

10. A 30 year old male patient came to you to consult you as the approximal-occlusal amalgam restoration you placed recently has undergone bulk fracture. What is the most likely factor to have caused this?
    - A. The amalgam was too deep (>1.5 mm in depth)
    - **B. The internal axio-pulpal line angle was too sharp**
    - C. The cavo-surface angle was 90o
    - D. Retention grooves were placed in the gingival floor of the cavity preparation

11. You have decided to use the selective etch technique while restoring tooth no 11 by using composite restoration. Which tooth structure should undergo etching with phosphoric acid?
    - A. the enamel and dentine
    - B. the dentine not overlying the pulp
    - **C. the enamel**
    - D. the glass ionomer restoration lining the cavity

12. You arc instructed to prepare a cavity for complex amalgam restoration in tooth no 46. You are placing addition retentive features in this cavity preparation. All of the following are the features of additional means of retention *except*
    - A. placement of an undercut box in the dentine
    - **B. indirect techniques**
    - C. a bonded amalgam restoration
    - D. dentine pins

13. At what age is calcification of the maxillary incisors and canines complete?
    - **A. 7 years**
    - B. 4 years
    - C. 5 years
    - D. 6 years

14. You are undergoing a direct pulp capping in tooth no 34.Regarding direct pulp capping which of the following is true
    A. Direct pulp capping can still take place if there is continued bleeding
    B. Direct pulp capping is when a protective dressing is placed over a small (<1mm2) pulpal exposure
    C. Direct pulp capping procedures can be used successfully in primary teeth
    D. The anti-bacterial properties of the dressing used in direct pulp capping will eliminate contamination of the exposed pulp

15. A 20 years old patient is presented to you in operative clinics complaining of dentin hypersensitivity. Regarding dentin hypersensitivity which of the following statement is correct
    A. Dentine hypersensitivity does not result from a routine scale and polish
    B. Treatments using potassium-containing toothpastes have been shown to lack subjective benefit when assessed
    C. Management may involve tubular exposure and nerve desensitisation
    D. Patients with tooth wear are not at increased risk of dentine hypersensitivity

16. In composite restoration the high is the C-factor the higher will be the polymerization shrinkage. Which of the following cavity design will have the highest C-factor?
    A. Class IV cavity
    B. Class II cavity in a premolar tooth
    C. Class II cavity in a molar tooth E A wide Class I cavity in a molar tooth
    D. A narrow Class I cavity in a molar tooth

17. Regarding composite and ceramics which of the following statement is true

A. Laboratory-processed composite restorations wear more than ceramics
B. Laboratory-processed composites wear more than direct composites
C. Ceramics wear more than direct composites
D. There is no clinically important difference in the wear between enamel, direct composites, ceramics and laboratory-processed composites

18. A 20 years old patient presented to you with proximal caries in tooth no 34. You decided to restore the cavity with bonded amalgam. Regarding bonded amalgam which of the following statement is true
    A. is highly cost-effective
    B. has insufficient evidence of improved retention over 2 years
    C. B significantly improved the marginal adaptation
    D. C significantly improved the post-operative sensitivity

19. You are restoring a cavity with resin composite restoration. How long is the 37% phosphoric acid gel usually left on the enamel before the application of self-etching primer?
    A. 5 seconds
    B. 15 seconds
    C. 30 seconds
    D. 1 minute

20. You are examining a patient with delayed eruption of maxillary first molar. Normally the maxillary first molar erupts into the oral cavity at the age of
    A. 9–10 years
    B. 7–8 years
    C. 6–7 years
    D. 2.5–3 years

21. You are restoring a class 11 Cavity with composite restoration. You decided to use a three stage total etch adhesive system. What is a three stage total etch adhesive system?
    A. It is a self-etching adhesive system
    B. A technique where the dentinal smear layer is dissolved by etchant followed by placement of primer and bonding resin
    C. A technique where the smear layer is removed by an etchant, followed by placement of a hydrophobic primer/resin combination
    D. It involves a selective etch of enamel, dentine and affected dentine

22. A 25 years old patient presented to you with occlusal caries in tooth no 46. You chose to restore the tooth with high copper amalgam. High copper amalgams have improved corrosion resistant properties over conventional amalgam alloys. This is due to the
    A. presence of the silver-tin alloy
    B. the high content of the silver-mercury $\gamma 1$ phase
    C. absence of galvanic currents E reduced plaque formation around high copper amalgam
    D. the absence of the tin-mercury $\gamma 2$ phase

23. While excavating caries from tooth no 45 in a 25 years old patient, you end up with a discolored tertiary dentin on the pulpal floor. The tertiary dentin is
    A. The dentine that is first deposited when the tooth is formed
    B. Dentine produced by either odontoblasts or subodontoblastic progenitor cells in response to noxious stimuli
    C. Peritubular dentine
    D. Intertubular dentine

24. You are presented with a 30 years old patient having proximal caries in tooth no 26. While preparing the cavity you decided to place grooves for additional retention. Grooves placed in the interproximal box of a class II amalgam restoration should be
    A. positioned at the enamel-dentine junction
    B. positioned 0.5 mm deep to the enamel-dentine junction
    C. positioned in the enamel
    D. D positioned 1.0 mm deep to the enamel-dentine junction

25. Loose enamel rods at the gingival floor of a class II amalgam cavity should be removed using
    A. Straight chisel
    B. Hatchet
    C. Gingival curetla
    D. **Gingival marginal trimmer**

26. What is the cavo-surface angle of prep for amalgam restoration?
    A. 30 degree
    B. 60 degree
    C. **90 degree**
    D. 130 degree

27. Hand instrument which we used to make internal angles retentive grooves and preparation of cavity walls in the cavity is
    A. **Angle former**
    B. Chisel
    C. File
    D. Enamel hatched

28. At which of the following locations on a mandibular molar do you complete the excavation of caries first
    A. Axial walls
    B. Pulpal floor over the mesial pulp horns
    C. Peripheral caries
    D. All of the above are correct

29. Which of the following materials has been shown to simulate reparative dentine formation most effectively when applied to the pulpal wall of a very deep cavity
    A. Copalite varnish
    B. **Calcium hydroxide preparation**
    C. Zinc phosphate cement
    D. Anhydrous glass ionomer cement

30. Clinical failure of the amalgam restoration usually occurs from
    A. Improper cavity preparation
    B. Faulty manipulation
    C. Both of the above
    D. None of the above

31. When polishing the amalgam restoration
    A. Avoid heat generation by using wet polishing paste
    B. Wait 24 hours
    C. **A and B**
    D. B only

32. A 20 years old patient came to your clinic. This patient had MOD amalgam restoration with deep mesial box, patient come with pain related to it after 1 month due to
    A. Pulp involvement
    B. Supraocclusion
    C. Upon contact
    D. Gingival recession

33. The x- ray of choice to detect the proximal caries of the anterior teeth is
    A. Periapical x-ray
    B. Bitewing x-ray
    C. Occlusal x-ray
    D. None of the above.

34. What is the copper ratio that eliminates gamma phase 2?
    A. 2% copper
    B. 4% copper
    C. 10% copper
    D. 13% copper

35. To prevent discoloration under amalgam filling
    A. Use Zn phosphate box
    B. Use cavity varnish
    C. Wash the cavity with NaOCl before filling
    D. Use the correct amalgam-alloy ratio

36. Patient complains of pain during mastication which had gold onlays. The pain could be due to
    A. Chemicals from cement
    B. High thermal conductivity of gold
    C. Related to periodontal ligament
    D. Cracked tooth or fractured surface

37. (7 days) after amalgam restoration, Patient came complaining of pain during putting spoon on the restored tooth because of
    A. Irreversible pulpitis
    B. Reversible pulpitis
    C. Broken amalgam
    D. Galvanic action

38. Bitewing radiograph is used to diagnose all the conditions *except*
    A. Proximal caries
    B. Secondary caries
    C. Gingival status
    D. Periapical abscess

39. Patient suffering from a cracked enamel, his chief complaint is pain on
    A. Hot stimuli
    B. Cold stimuli
    C. A&B
    D. Electric test

40. At which location in enamel is the density of enamel crystals is the lowest
    A. Prismless enamel
    B. DEJ
    C. Center of enamel Prisms
    D. Edge of enamel Prisms

41. Pins are inserted into
    A. Enamel
    B. Dentin
    C. Enamel and dentin (DEJ)
    D. Any of the above

42. Incipient caries is diagnosed by
    A. Fiber optic light
    B. Tactile examination
    C. X-ray film
    D. Electrical conduction

43. One week after filling of class II restoration, the Patient presents with a complaint of tenderness on mastication and bleeding from the gingival. The dentist should initially
    A. Check the occlusion
    B. Check the contract area
    C. Consider the probability of hyperemia
    D. Explain to the Patient that the retainer irritated the surrounding soft tissue and prescribe ananalgesic and warm oral rinse

44. Which one of the following is not a characteristic of dentinal hypersensitivity?
    A. It is one of the most successfully treated chronic dental problems
    B. Its prevalence range from 8 to 30%
    C. The majority of the Patients who experience it are from 20 to 40 years of age
    D. One source of the irritation that leads to hypersensitivity is improper tooth brushing

45. A Patient 25years old come to dental clinic complaining from discoloration of his teeth. By clinical examination there is white opaque mottling enamel the possible cause of discoloration is
    A. Enamel hypocalcification
    B. Enamel fluorosis
    C. Enamel hypoplasia
    D. Amelogenesis imperfect

46. Patient 35years old come to dental clinic complaining from fracture amalgam restoration in lower first molar by clinical examination there is isthmus fracture the cause of fracture is
    A. Improper resistance form of cavity
    B. Inadequate retention at proximal portion
    C. Improper outline form of cavity
    D. Improper convenience form of cavity

47. Patient come to dental clinic with multiple white spot lesions the possible line of treatment is
    A. Composite resin restoration
    B. Glass-ionmer restoration
    C. Remineralization
    D. Composite glass-ionmer sandwich technique

48. A teen-aged patient presents with numerous proximal carious lesions that undermine the occlusal enamel. Which of the following is the treatment-of choice?
    A. Restore involved teeth with onlays to preserve occlusion
    B. Restore involved teeth as rapidly as possible using dental amalgam
    C. Place the patient on a prevention regimen and delay treatment until the effectiveness of home care is evaluated
    D. Restore involved teeth with crown to preserve occlusion

49. Your patient fractured the distal incisal edge of tooth #9 there are no caries or existing restorations. The tooth needs restoration with a class IV composite. List the major steps you need to accomplish before placement of the restorative material
    A. Clean the surface of the tooth
    B. Select shade
    C. Place the rubber dam (isolate)
    D. Bevel the margins (prepare the tooth)

50. A patient has sensitivity in a mandibular premolar. A well-condensed Class V dental amalgam restoration was placed in the tooth five months previously, with no discomfort for the first four months. Since then, it has become painful. The problem probably relates to
    A. Marginal leakage
    B. Toothbrush abrasion
    C. A fractured restoration
    D. Irreversible pulpal damage

51. Which of the following statements correctly describes the relationship between marginal leakage of an amalgam restoration and age of the restoration?
    A. Marginal leakage increases as the restoration ages
    B. Marginal leakage decreases as the restoration ages

C. Marginal leakage is severe throughout the life of the restoration

D. Marginal leakage does not exist throughout the life of the restoration

52. Total etching adhesive systems means

A. Adhesive systems never using an acid etching as a first step

B. Adhesive systems using an acid etching as a first step

C. Adhesive systems using acid + primer as first step before application of bonding

D. Agent adhesive systems using an acid etching as a second step

53. Main problems of composite resins restorations are the following *except*

A. Water sorption and polymerization shrinkage

B. High thermal coefficient of expansion and low wear resistance

C. Discoloration

D. Chemical union and adhesion

54. Nature of adhesion and union between glass ionomer cements and tooth structures are

A. Mechanical union

B. **Chemical union and adhesion**

C. Macro-mechanical union

D. Micro-mechanical

55. Which of the following faults in class II restorations may be predisposing factors to periodontal disease?

A. Gingival overhang

B. Weak proximal contact

C. Broad contact faciolingually

D. Improperly shaped occlusal embrasure

56. A bevel contraindicated on the cavosurface angles of a class I dental amalgam cavity preparation. Which of the following best explains why?
    - A. This type of margin is prone to microleakage
    - B. The cavosurface bevel makes burnishing more difficult
    - **C. A thin flange of the amalgam restorative material might fracture**
    - D. As the tooth undergoes natural attrition, the amalgam margin can abrade

57. The occlusal isthmus of an MO dental amalgam restoration is more resistant to fracture if the
    - A. Pulpal depth is 1mm
    - B. Occlusal dovetail is present
    - C. **Axiopulpal line angle is rounded**
    - D. Unsupported enamel at the gingiva cavosurface margin is planned

58. When using the acid etch technique to restore a class IV fracture, exposed dentin should first be covered with
    - A. Cavity varnish
    - B. Phosphoric acid
    - C. **A calcium hydroxide liner**
    - D. Zinc oxide-eugenol cement

59. A 30-year-old patient came to the clinic with brownish discoloration of all his teeth (intrinsic discoloration) & yellowish in U/V light the most likely cause is
    - A. Fluorosis
    - **B. Tetracycline**
    - C. Amelogensis imperfect
    - D. Dentogensis imperfectea

60. The specific purposes of acid etching of enamel before insertion of a composite restoration is to provide
    - A. A dry surface
    - B. Less surface area
    - **C. More surface area**
    - D. A roughened surface

61. Patient 20years old came to dental clinic complaining from stain. On clinical examination this stain is found to be extrinsic yellowish brown stains. The possible cause of stains is
    - A. Enamel hypocalcification
    - **B. Accumulation of plaque and calculus**
    - C. Enamel hypoplasia
    - D. Enamelogenes is imperfect

62. 30-year-old patient came to dental clinic complaining from sensitivity in lower first molar amalgam restoration. On clinical examination there is caries around the margin of the restoration, cause of sensitivity is
    - **A. Recurrent caries**
    - B. Inadequate retention at proximal portion
    - C. Improper outline form of cavity
    - D. Improper convenience form of cavity

63. Patient came to dental clinic complaining of teeth with multiple white spot lesions, possible line of treatment is
    - A. Composite resin restoration
    - B. Glass-ionmer restoration
    - **C. Remineralization**
    - D. Composite glass-ionmer sandwich technique

64. A teenaged patient presents with numerous proximal and occlusal carious lesions that undermine the occlusal enamel. Which of the following is the treatment-of choice?
    A. Restore involved teeth with onlays to preserve occlusion
    B. Restore involved teeth as rapidly as possible using dental amalgam
    C. Place the patient on a prevention regimen and delay treatment until the effectiveness of home care is evaluated
    D. Restore involved teeth with crown to preserve occlusion

65. Your patient fractured the mesial incisal edge of tooth #8 there are no caries or existing restorations. The tooth needs restoration with a class IV composite. List the major steps you need to accomplish before placement of the restorative material.
    A. Clean the surface of the tooth
    B. Select shade
    C. Place the rubber dam (isolate)
    D. Bevel the margins (prepare the tooth)

66. A patient has sensitivity in maxillary premolar. A well-made Class V composite restoration was placed in the tooth five months previously, with no discomfort for the first four months. Since then, it has become painful. The problem probably relates to
    A. Marginal leakage
    B. Toothbrush abrasion
    C. A fractured restoration
    D. Irreversible pulpal damage

67. Patient came to dental clinic with brown staining after several week of use mouth rinse, possible cause is
    A. Composite resin restoration
    B. Glass-ionomer restoration
    C. Remineralization
    D. Chlorhexidine mouth rinse

68. 35-year-old patient came to dental clinic complaining from fractured amalgam restoration in lower second molar. On clinical examination of fracture, possible cause is
    A. Improper resistance form
    B. Improper retention form
    C. Over extension of the cavity preparation
    D. Under extension of the cavity preparation

69. Patient has proximal amalgam restoration in lower second premolars since five years. He is complaining from pain. On clinical and radiographical examination there is marginal leakage between tooth and the restoration. Which of the following statement determine the marginal leakage of an amalgam restoration and age of the restoration?
    A. Marginal leakage increases as the restoration ages
    B. Marginal leakage decreases as the restoration ages
    C. Marginal leakage is severe throughout the life of the restoration
    D. Marginal leakage does not exist throughout the life of the restoration

70. During removal of caries in lower first molar the disto-buccal cusp is undermined by caries, the best line of treatment is
    A. Removal of distobuccal cusp
    B. Leave the distobuccal cusp
    C. Removed the disto-buccal cusp and doing cusp capping
    D. Removed the disto-buccal cusp and without doing cusp capping

71. Patient has composite restoration in upper central incisors and complaining from change in colour, possible cause is
    A. Bulk discoloration
    B. Marginal discoloration
    C. Surface discoloration
    D. Moture contamination

72. Patient came to dental clinic with non cavitated carious teeth. The best and the most conservative line of treatment is
    A. Remineralization of the teeth
    B. Using pit and fissure sealant
    C. Restoration of the teeth
    D. Removal of plaque

73. During clinical examination, many patients in a dental clinic had non cavitated initial inter proximal caries, best line of treatment is
    A. Ion resin infiltration system
    B. Pit and fissure sealant
    C. Glass-ionomer restoration
    D. Composite resin restoration

74. 50-year-old patient complain from pain in lower second molar. On clinical examination there is cavitated root caries, possible line of treatment is
    A. Composite resin restoration
    B. Amalgam restoration
    C. Glass-ionmer restoration
    D. Cast gold restoration

75. Adult patient who has stains on his teeth want to get it removed. On clinical examination this stain is found to be extrinsic and yellowish brown, due to accumulation of plaque and calculus. Possible line of treatment is
    A. Bleaching
    B. Micro abrasion
    C. Scaling and polishing
    D. Ozone therapy

76. A 25 years old patient presented to you for composite restoration in the anterior teeth. You decided to use vita classical (Lumin Vacuum) shade tabs for the correct colour for the composite restoration. Which of the following represent the correct order of the tabs in the highest to lowest value (or brightness)?
    A. B1, B2, A1,D2,A2 AND C1
    B. B1,A1,B1,D2,A2 AND C1
    C. B1,A1,B2,D2,A2 AND C1
    D. B1,A1, C1B2,D2, AND A2

77. A 30 years old patient presented to you for restoration. You planned to use polycorboxlate cement as a temporary dressing. Which of these substances is not usually a constituent of the material during mixing?
    A. Zinc Oxide
    B. Water
    C. Polyacylic acid
    D. Eugenol

78. While restoring a class II cavity in mandibular molar you preferred to use high copper amalgam as a restorative material. High copper amalgam have improved corrosion resistance over conventional alloy, due to
    A. The high content of silver mercury phase
    B. Presence of silver tin alloy
    C. The absence of tin mercury phase
    D. Reduce plaque formation around high copper amalgam

79. A 50 years old patient came to your dental surgery with a deformed amalgam restoration in maxillary molar. You noticed a marginal failure in the restoration which could be due to creep in amalgam. Creep can be defined as
    A. Ductility
    B. The flexural strength of a material

C. **The time dependent permanent deformation under an applied load**
D. The rigidity of a material

80. A 20 years old patient came to you with pits and fissure caries in the mandibular molars. In treatment planning you decided, preventive resin restorations. Regarding preventive resin restoration in mandibular molars, which of the following is true?
    A. Any carious dentin can be treated with fluoride varnish
    B. The fissures are routinely reduced to a depth of 1.5mm
    C. **Any carious dentin underlying the fissure is removed**
    D. Any carious dentin underlying the fissure is sealed with Glass-ionomer

81. A 15 years old patient presented to you with poor oral hygiene and multiple class V cavities. A class v cavity is found on the
    A. Occlusal surface of a tooth
    B. Interproximal surface of a tooth
    C. Incisal surface of a tooth
    D. **Cervical third of buccal and lingual surface of a tooth**

82. A 16 years old patient presented to you with multiple carious lesions. On history taking you noticed that the patient has, poor dietary habits and he frequently take sugary snakes in between meals. What is the critical pH of enamel?
    A. pH2.5
    B. **pH5.5**
    C. pH3.5
    D. pH1.5

83. A 35 years old patient presented to you with grossly carious vital mandibular first molar. While cavity preparation you decided to uses dentinal pins for increased retention of the amalgam restoration. Regarding dentinal pins which of the following is true
    A. A hole minimum of 4 mm is placed in the dentin

B. A minimum of 1 mm of amalgam is necessary to cover the pin
C. Bending pins will not fracture dentin
D. The self-threaded pin is the most retentive type of pin

84. A 23 Years old patient presented to you with a grossly carious vital mandibular first molar. You decided to make ceramic onlay, what is the minimum amount of cuspal reduction for ceramic onlay?
A. 0.5mm
B. 1.0mm
C. 1.5mm
D. 2mm

85. A 55 years old patient presented to you with proximal caries in maxillary first molar. You planned to make a class II cavity in the tooth and decided to place grooves in the proximal box. Grooves placed in the proximal box of class II amalgam restoration should be
A. Position in the enamel
B. Positioned at enamel-dentin junction
C. Positioned 0.5 mm deep to enamel-dentin junction
D. Positioned 2 mm deep to enamel-dentin junction

86. You are preparing a class 11 cavity in maxillary first molar in a 45 years old patient. As a rule, when operating in the maxillary arch,
A. the maxillary occlusal surfaces should be oriented approximately parallel to the floor
B. the maxillary occlusal surfaces should be oriented approximately 45 degrees to the floor
C. the maxillary occlusal surfaces should be oriented approximately 60 degrees to the floor
D. the maxillary occlusal surfaces should be oriented approximately perpendicular to the floor

87. A 25 years old patient presented to you with fractured MOD amalgam restoration in tooth no 46. In treatment planning you decided to replace

the amalgam restoration. All of the following modifications will be done in the tooth preparation to prevent future fracture of the restoration. *except*

A. Divergent walls
B. Box shape
C. Inclusion of weakened tooth structure
D. Preservation of cusps and marginal ridges

88. You are making a Mesio-occlusal cavity preparation (class II) for amalgam restoration. What cavosurface angle will you place during this cavity preparation for amalgam restoration?

A. 90 degrees
B. 50 degrees
C. 70 degrees
D. 110 degrees

89. You have been asked to make an ideal class I cavity preparation for amalgam restoration on tooth # 36. The pulpal floor for this cavity should be

A. In the enamel
B. At the DEJ
C. 0.2 mm inside the DEJ
D. 1.5 mm inside the DEJ

90. You are making a Class I cavity preparation on the tooth # 16. During the cavity preparation all of the following can determine the location of cavity outline form *except*

A. Extent of caries
B. Presence of unsupported enamel
C. Depth of the lesion
D. Occlusal contact

91. A patient came to you with carious lesion involving occluso-lingual surface of tooth no 16.The outline form for occluso-lingual (OL) cavity preparation in tooth no 16 should be

A. One third of the lingual surface
B. One half of the lingual surface
C. The length of the fissure
D. One fourth of the lingual surface

92. A 25 years old young male came in your clinic with multiple carious teeth. After the clinical examination you have decided to do full mouth radiographic survey. How many radiographs are required for full mouth examination?
    A. 6 bitewings and 14 periapical film
    B. 4 bitewings and 12 periapical films
    C. 4 bitewings and 18 periapical films
    D. 6 bitewing and 12 periapical films

93. A 16 years old girl came to you with the complaint of sensitivity to hot and cold on the right side of her mouth. Clinical and radiographic examination revealed the carious lesion on the occlusal surface of tooth no 16. During the cavity preparation for an amalgam restoration the crossing of the oblique ridge in the tooth no 16 is permissible in all *except*
    A. When the ridge has a deep fissure
    B. When the ridge is undermined with caries
    C. When it is necessary for retention
    D. In incipient caries in mesial and distal pit

94. A 20 years old patient presented in your clinic with multiple cervical lesions in the upper anterior teeth. You have decided to place the caries control restorations by using the glass ionomer cement. It possesses all of the following properties *except*
    A. It is well tolerated by the pulp
    B. It does not remain rigid under the load
    C. It releases fluoride ions to the tooth structure
    D. It adheres chemically to enamel and dentin

95. A 23 years old patient presented with a deep carious lesion on the cervical one third of tooth no 43. You have decided to restore this tooth by using a sandwich technique. Regarding the sandwich technique which of the following statement is not true
    A. The glass ionomer material bonds both to the tooth structure and composite
    B. Fluoride contained in the glass-ionomer material reduces the potential for recurrent caries
    C. The glass-ionomer material because of its bond to tooth structure provides a better seal when used at non-enamel margins
    D. The glass-ionomer material because of its weak bond to non-enamel margins increases recurrent caries

96. In a 24 years old male patient you are restoring an extensive class II cavity by using an Automatrix system. It is a
    A. It is a universal matrix system
    B. Retainer less matrix system
    C. Toffemire matrix system
    D. Ivory matrix system

97. A 27 year old patient presented with an extensive decay with cuspal loss on the lingual surface in tooth no 46. You have decided to restore this tooth with amalgam and self- threading pins. The optimum depth of a self- threading pin for an amalgam restoration is
    A. 0.5 mm
    B. 2 mm
    C. 1 mm
    D. 5 mm

98. A 50 year old patient came with pain and sensitivity on the lower left side of his face. On clinical examination you have found an old fractured amalgam restoration in tooth no 47. Most common fracture occurring in amalgam restoration is seen at

A. The contact area
B. The isthmus area
C. Cavosurface margin
D. Gingival floor

99. In 18 year old patient, you have placed a glass ionomer restoration in tooth no 26. The final finishing of this glass ionomer restoration will be done after
    A. 24 hours
    B. 7 ½ minutes
    C. 30 minutes
    D. 1 hour

100. A 28 years old patient came to your clinic with a badly decayed tooth no 37. You have decided to place an amalgam restoration by capping the cusps. Regarding the cusp capping which of the following statement is true
    A. Cusp reduction usually is mandatory when the outline form has extended one-thirds the distance from a primary groove to a cusp tip
    B. Cusp reduction usually is mandatory when the outline form has extended one- fourth the distance from a primary groove to a cusp tip
    C. Cusp reduction usually is mandatory when the outline form has extended two-fifth the distance from a primary groove to a cusp tip
    D. Cusp reduction usually is mandatory when the outline form has extended two-thirds the distance from a primary groove to a cusp tip

101. While restoring a Class II cavity preparation on tooth no 36, you are applying Tofflemire matrix and you are facing difficulty in passing the matrix band between teeth no 36 and 37. The thickness of the band for Tofflemire matrix system should be
   A. 0.01mm to 0.05mm
   B. 1mm to 2mm
   C. 0.025mm to 0.05mm
   D. 0.05mm to 1mm

102. While restoring the upper right posterior teeth with composite in a 24 years old young lady, you have placed the rubber dam for isolation. Rubber dam inversion with knot ligature is mostly indicated when the tooth preparation margins are
   A. Supra-gingival
   B. Below the epithelial insertion
   C. Equigingival
   D. Above the epithelial insertion

103. A 29 years old lady came to your clinic with class V cavities in most of his posterior teeth because of occlusal trauma (Abfraction). You have decided to restore these cavities with composite. Which composite chemistry is indicated for the restoration of these cavities?
   A. Low matrix content with high filler content
   B. Low matrix content with low filler content
   C. Matrix and filler content can be equal
   D. Higher matrix content with low filler content

104. A 60 years old patient presented to your clinic with multiple root caries lesion in posterior teeth due to poor manual dexterity. You have planned to restore these lesions with amalgam. Which of the following tooth preparation design is best for these restorations?
   A. Box only preparation
   B. Tunnel preparation
   C. Slot preparation
   D. Modified tooth preparation

REFERENCES

Avijit Banaerjee; 2015. *Pickard Guide to Minimal Invasive Operative Dentistry.*

Edwin Kidd; 2016. *Essential of Dental Caries.*

Freedman, George A; 2013. *Contemporary Esthetic Dentistry.*

James B Summit; 2013. *Summit Fundamental of Operative Dentistry, A Contemporary Approach.*

Lussi, Adrian; 2012. *Advances in Restorative Dentistry.*

Theodore M, Harald O, Edward J; 2012. *Sturdevant's Art and Science of Operative Dentistry.*

In: Scenario Based MCQ in Dentistry ISBN: 978-1-53617-298-0
Editors: M. Khursheed Alam et al.

Chapter 6

SCENARIO BASED MCQS IN ENDODONTICS

Ravi Jothish, MDS and Shilpa S. Magar, MDS
Department of Conservative Dentistry & Endodontics,
College of Dentistry, Jouf University, Aljouf, Saudi Arabia

The art and science of endodontics have traversed an amazing journey since the day it saved the patient from the evil hands of the extractionists. Science has helped this discipline to save teeth with predictable success while the clinician performs the art of healing. Advances in material science and technology and tons of dedicated, meticulous research has catapulted endodontics into a never before paradigm.

Over the next few pages an attempt has been made to capture a gist of this eventful journey even though it is difficult to cover all the aspects of endodontics. Pathology of pulp and periapical tissues lay the foundation for this venture and provides an insight into the diagnostic tools and recent advancements. Special attention has been given to the materials used and how they have evolved over the years from cork and wood shavings to arsenic and molten metal and eventually to adhesive obturation, MTA and bioceramics. Sincere attempt has been made to capture the story behind the evolution of concepts from hollow tube and mountain pass to monobloc theory. Evolution of root canal instruments and instrumentation techniques are also briefly discussed through the chapter. Sometimes non-surgical endodontics fails despite providing standard care. Magnification and latest advances in imaging have almost succeeded in finding the reason for such failures. An effort has been put to present these matters so as to encourage critical thinking on diagnosis and their evidence based management. In a nut shell, this chapter provides an overview of the discipline of endodontics and effective tool for a round of rapid revision.

1. A 64-year-old woman who had an endodontic appointment a day back, reported at the clinic seeking an emergency appointment. She presented with distension of the left suborbital region with ptosis of the eye and loss of Naso-labial fold. Facial swelling lacked redness, was painless but had marked crepitus. As a clinician, your diagnosis would be
   - A. Allergic reactions
   - **B. Emphysema**
   - C. Hematoma
   - D. Angioneurotic edema

2. A 52-year-old woman reported at the endodontic clinic for an emergency appointment. She had swelling on right side of her face which apparently extends to the right submandibular and sublingual regions on the affected side. She had bluish red bruises all over the swelling, difficulty in opening her right eye and limited mouth opening but no paraesthesia. She informs the dentist that she was root canal treated 3 days back by the neighbourhood GP and that she had severe pain even as she was getting anesthetized by the GP; pain has not subsided ever since despite taking painkillers. The endodontist reassured her and suggested antibiotics and warm compresses and oral rinses in addition to the painkiller. She was advised to come for a review after 3 days; the most likely diagnosis for this patient is

A. Hematoma
B. Domestic abuse
C. Emphysema
D. Sodium hypochlorite accident

3. An 8-year-old boy with a broken upper anterior tooth was brought to dental clinic. Boy had an unfortunate accident 12 hours back in which the upper left central incisor was broken. On examination dentist could see pinpoint exposure of pulp; bleeding had stopped at the time of inspection. Periapical radiograph ruled out complicated crown and root fracture. Considering the findings and the best possible prognosis, the initial treatment for this fractured tooth is most likely to be
   A. Pulp capping
   B. Partial pulpotomy
   C. Full pulpotomy
   D. Pulpectomy

4. A 9-year-old boy with a broken upper central incisor was brought to dental clinic. He had an unfortunate fall 4 days back. After clinical and radiographic examination, the dentist decided to perform pulpectomy and initiate an apexification procedure. What could be the most probable reason for this treatment plan?
   A. Incomplete root formation of the concerned tooth
   B. Inability to seal after pulpotomy
   C. Prognosis of pulpotomy is poor
   D. Tooth structure is too compromised for any vital pulp therapies

5. An endodontist decided to perform pulpectomy and apexification on an 8 year old boy with a broken upper left central incisor. Which among the following is not a prime consideration during this treatment?
   A. Status of the pulp
   B. Susceptibility of the tooth to fracture
   C. Use of appropriate filling material
   D. Formation of an apical stop

6. A 25-year-old youth met with road traffic accident and was brought to a dental clinic. He had minor soft tissue laceration; on intraoral examination upper right lateral incisor was found to exhibit some luxation. No external fracture lines were detected. But periapical radiograph shows a minor middle third fracture of the root. After thorough examination; the dentist decided to give semi rigid splint for the tooth. Under which condition may the dentist consider a future root canal treatment on that tooth?
    A. Healing with calcified tissue
    B. Healing with interproximal connective tissue
    C. Healing with interproximal bone and connective tissue
    D. Interproximal inflammatory tissue without healing

7. A 22-year-old patient consulted his dentist complaining of discoloured teeth and increase in sensitivity. Multiple teeth with brownish and yellowish-brown discoloration were found. Local pitting and generalised thinning of enamel was observed, but all teeth responded positively to vitality tests. He mentioned that his milk teeth also had similar discoloration. There is no relevant family history. Bleaching was suggested by the dentist as initial treatment. The condition is most likely to be
    A. Focal hypocalcification
    B. Amelogenesis imperfecta
    C. Dentinogenesis Imperfecta
    D. Endemic fluorosis

8. A 27-year-old male patient reported at the local health centre complaining of broken teeth and poor appearance. The physician who attended him referred him to the consultant dentist in the centre. On examination he was found to have multiple discoloured teeth which were found to be very brittle. Discoloration varied from yellowish brown to greyish blue to deep amber. On further questioning it was found that his milk teeth also had similar problem. Meanwhile the physician's report mentioned that patient is suffering from brittle

bones. The dentist suggested multiple root canal treatment followed by comprehensive rehabilitation. What is he suffering from?

A. Erythroblastosis foetalis
B. Amelogenesis Imperfecta
C. Dentinogenesis Imperfecta
D. Dentin dysplasia

9. Major aim of root canal therapy is address apical periodontitis by disinfecting and sealing the canal. In the past, this was achieved by 'Cleaning and shaping'; but now the usage has changed to 'shaping and cleaning'. What does this signify?
   A. Modern endodontic instruments first shape and then clean.
   B. Modern endodontic instruments shapes more, cleans less
   C. Shaping the canal is more important than cleaning.
   D. Shaping facilitate cleaning action of irrigants

10. A 24-year-old man had an unfortunate fall; his left upper central incisor got avulsed. Patient does not have any associated head injury and is fully conscious. There was no immediate dental care available in his vicinity. What would be the best thing to do considering the long term prognosis of the tooth?
    A. Place the tooth in his buccal vestibule and take him to a dental clinic as early as possible
    B. Place tooth in milk and take him to a dental clinic as early as possible
    C. Place tooth in sterile container and take him to a dental clinic as early as possible
    D. Place tooth in tap water and take him to dental clinic as early as possible

11. A 12-year-old boy had an unfortunate fall while playing in his school; his right upper central incisor got avulsed. He was attended by a physician in the school dispensary who ruled out any associated head injury. The boy is fully conscious now. There was no immediate dental

care available in his vicinity. What would be the best thing to do considering the long term prognosis of the tooth?

A. Place the tooth in his buccal vestibule and take him to a dental clinic as early as possible

B. Place tooth in milk and take him to a dental clinic as early as possible

C. Place tooth in sterile container and take him to a dental clinic as early as possible

D. Place tooth in tap water and take him to dental clinic as early as possible

12. A 40-year-old woman visited her neighbourhood dentist complaining of a broken tooth. On examination lower right first molar was found to be fractured. The tooth having a complex amalgam restoration was found to be root canal treated 7 years back. Which among the following is the most possible reason for the fracture?

A. Plastic deformation of dentin

B. Brittility following moisture loss

C. Loss of root vitality weakened the tooth

D. Destruction of its coronal structure

13. A 25-year-old man met with a road accident and was brought to the nearby hospital. After ruling out any significant head injury, he was referred to the dental consultation for a check-up. No significant findings were found except for mild lip laceration and minor bruises on his forehead. Radiograph showed apical third fracture of a maxillary central incisor, but without any mobility. The most generally accepted treatment for this tooth is

A. Extraction of the tooth

B. Frequent pulp testing and radiographic examination

C. Immediate pulp extirpation

D. Splinting the tooth with orthodontic band and sectional arch wire.

14. A 17-year-old boy had an unfortunate fall while playing football in college. There was no significant injury, except for mild lip laceration and a minor Ellis Class 1 fracture of left lateral incisor. Radiograph showed apical third fracture of the tooth without any mobility. After treatment the tooth would most likely
    A. Exhibit ankylosis
    B. Exhibit external resorption and gradually exfoliate
    C. Exhibit internal resorption
    D. Remain vital and functional

15. Permanent maxillary central incisor of an 8-year-old boy is discoloured and was found to have a mid-crown fracture. The parent informed that he had a minor fall several months back but did not approach the dentist since he was asymptomatic. The tooth did not respond to pulp vitality test and was found to be necrotic. Periapical radiograph revealed an incompletely formed root with open apex. Treatment of choice is
    A. Formocresol pulpotomy
    B. Calcium hydroxide pulpotomy
    C. Root Canal Therapy
    D. Pulpectomy followed by apexification

16. Eight-year-old Farhan fell down and got his central incisor avulsed 20 minutes back. The avulsed tooth was picked up from the ground and found to be contaminated with debris. Child was rushed to the nearby dental clinic, immediate treatment given is
    A. Clean root surface with saline rinse and implant
    B. Clean and curette the root surface before implant
    C. Clean root surface, perform RCT and implant
    D. Scrub the root surface thoroughly and implant

17. A 45-year-old female reported at the dental clinic complaining of pain in relation to right lower first molar. There are no significant clinical or radiographic findings except that pain appears when bite is released after biting down on hard objects. What could be the cause of this pain?
    A. Impacted right third molar
    B. Maxillary sinusitis
    C. Cracked tooth
    D. Severe periodontitis

18. A 54-year-old male reported at the dental clinic complaining of pain in relation to right lower first molar. There are no significant clinical or radiographic findings except that pain appears when bite is released after biting down on hard objects. What is the immediate treatment for this tooth?
    A. No treatment needed now; keep monitoring
    B. Band and stabilize the tooth with orthodontic band
    C. Relieve the occlusion and monitor
    D. Root canal treatment followed by full crown

19. During root canal treatment, the apical constriction is violated and enlarged to a size # 70 instrument. Which of the following is appropriate treatment or this canal?
    A. Fit a size # 70 GP cone with sealer but don't condense so as to keep the GP from being pushed into the foramen
    B. Reinstrument the canal 1mm short of the apex to a size # 80 and obturate
    C. Fit a size # 70 GP cone with sealer and carefully condense
    D. Obturate with GP and surgically remove extruded excess

20. The crown of a root canal treated premolar tooth is fractured near the gingival margin. The coronal end of the silver cone used for obturation is visible at that level. This tooth is managed best by
    A. Preparing post space alongside the silver cone

B. Removing the silver cone, make notches in it and then replace it in the canal with freshly mixed sealer; coronal part is removed
C. Grinding away the coronal part of the silver cone using round burs or end cutting burs
D. Removing the silver cone, retreating the canal using GP points and then preparing the post space.

21. Patient came next day after access opening of non-vital tooth with severe tenderness and swelling of that region. What could be the reason?
    A. Endodontic Flare-up
    B. Sodium Hypochlorite Accident
    C. Improper closed dressing
    D. Improper Diagnosis of tooth and wrong treatment

22. Patient complaining of swelling on lower right back tooth region since 6 months. Clinically Tooth showing with the Moderate deep caries, deep pocket, and tenderness to horizontal percussion. Swelling near the 46 which is fluctuant, laterally placed. Radiologically showing severe bone loss with respect to 46. On vitality test, the tooth showing positive response with heat and EPT. What should the diagnosis
    A. Acute apical abscess
    B. Acute periodontal abscess
    C. Acute irreversible pulpitis
    D. Apical periodontitis

23. If you want to do the endodontic treatment of tooth which have dilacerated root and also with curved canals, which method of biomechanical preparation you would prefer?
    A. Step back method
    B. Use of larger instruments with reaming action
    C. Contraindicated for endodontic treatment
    D. Crown down technique

24. A 40-year male patient awake with swollen face, oedema around eyes and upper lips with redness and dryness. On clinical examination shows deep silicate restoration in anterior teeth and no caries with same tooth. Thermal test, percussion and palpation are negative and radiological finding shows periapical area of rarefaction. Condition is
    A. Acute periapical abscess
    B. Angioneurotic edema
    C. Acute maxillary sinusitis
    D. Acute apical periodontitis

25. A cyst at the apex of an upper central incisor measuring 1 cm in diameter is visualized in radiograph and confirmed by aspiration biopsy. Which treatment you would prefer?
    A. Incision and drainage from the labial mucosa
    B. Extraction of tooth
    C. Do the endodontic treatment, followed by flap surgery to remove cystic Lesion
    D. Nonsurgical endodontic treatment

26. A 35-year-old patient came to clinic with the pain and swelling in upper right back tooth region. On clinical examination showing the temporary restoration with and mild tenderness on percussion. Patient has history of root canal done 4-5 days back. Radiological examination, showing the good Obturation without any periapical radiolucency. What should be the treatment?
    A. Endodontic Retreatment
    B. Apicoectomy
    C. No need any treatment only require follow up
    D. Prescribe mild analgesics and inform patient about possible discomfort for the first few days.

27. Patient complains of bleeding gums with 46 regions. On examination shows deep periodontal pocket with 46 but no caries and positive response with the thermal test. What should be first line of treatment?
    A. Need only periodontal treatment
    B. Need periodontal as well as endodontic treatment
    C. Poor prognosis advice for extraction
    D. Endodontic treatment

28. When you should decide whether a prepared root canal can be obturated following placement of an inter-appointment dressing?
    A. The tooth must not be associated with a fistula
    B. The tooth must be symptom-free
    C. The root canal space must be free of all bacteria
    D. Should be confirming by Microbiological testing only

29. When assessing a tooth to determine whether endodontics is a suitable treatment option, which of the following does NOT contraindicate endodontic treatment?
    A. Extensive subgingival caries
    B. The dentist lacks the necessary endodontic skills
    C. The tooth forms an abutment of a bridge
    D. The patient's attitude is unreceptive and unwilling to accept endodontic Treatment

30. During root canal treatment by mistake if you have separated the endodontic file in the middle third of a straight root canal. What should not be first further treatment option in removing a file?
    A. Attempt to remove the file with an endosonic tip
    B. Surgical removal of the separated file
    C. Using small files to remove or bypass the separated file
    D. Taking a radiograph to confirm the separation of the file and its position

31. Patient came to the clinic immediately after dental trauma on road accident with extruded upper right central incisor. What should be your first line of treatment?
    A. Advice radiograph
    B. Replace the tooth in its original position and follow up
    C. Leave it observe the tooth
    D. Inform the patient about consequences

32. A tooth with periapical radiolucency indicated for endodontic treatment, and you performed endodontic treatment with good obturation and good apical sealing. When you should be expected the size of periapical radiolucency reduces?
    A. Immediately after endodontic treatment
    B. Follow up after 1 year
    C. It depends on size of the periapical radiolucency
    D. does not response to reduce size of radiolucency after endodontic treatment

33. A 15-year-old patient came with the complaining of yellow discoloration of upper right central incisor. Patient giving history of trauma 5 years back and on radiologically tooth showing open apex. Thermal test is negative with respect to the involved tooth. What should be the best treatment option?
    A. Apexogenesis
    B. Apexification with MTA
    C. Surgical retrograde filling
    D. No need endodontic treatment wait till apex close

34. Patient came with the localized intraoral swelling with respect to #46. Which test you perform with the same tooth to differentiate between apical abscess and periodontal abscess?
    A. Radiograph
    B. Percussion test

C. Pulp Vitality test
D. Palpation

35. During root canal treatment, you have given intracanal dressing and closed the access with temporary restoration. Next day if patient came with the severe pain and swelling in same tooth, what you will do?
   A. Incision and drainage
   B. Replace the dressing and prescribe antibiotic
   C. Replace dressing with corticosteroids
   D. Remove dressing and keep open for some days before replace restoration

36. A 15-year-old boy fallen from bicycle 1 week ago and came to the clinic with broken central incisors after that accident. Clinically shows the pinpoint pulp exposure but tooth is vital. What you will do?
   A. Perform pulpectomy
   B. Pulpotomy
   C. Place calcium hydroxide and Composite restoration
   D. Calcium hydroxide pulpotomy

37. Patient came with severe pain while eating in endodontically treated tooth. Radiologically shows good Obturation. On history taking RCT done 1 year back and advised to go for Crown. But patient didn't get full crown. What you are suspecting for reason of severe pain?
   A. Vertical root fracture
   B. Horizontal root fracture
   C. Improper sealing of apex
   D. Improper coronal sealing

38. Patient wishes to remove discoloration of his endodontically treated anterior tooth. Patient is not ready for full jacket crown. What technique you prefer to remove this discoloration?
    - A. In-office Vital Bleaching
    - **B. Walking Bleach**
    - C. Home bleaching
    - D. Convince the patient for full jacket crown

39. Patient with pain in upper right tooth region, and the patient not able to locate the tooth cause pain. What is the least reliable way to do test pulp?
    - A. Heat test
    - **B. Electric pulp test**
    - C. Percussion test
    - D. Cold test

40. Patient complaining of draining pus with endo treated upper central incisor without pain. Radiograph is taken by GP tracing from sinus opening, and GP appearing in lateral side of root. What would be the reason for drainage?
    - A. Due to the periodontal abscess
    - B. Periodonitits
    - **C. Lateral accessory canal**
    - D. Fracture of tooth

41. A young, 12-year-old boy presents with reddish over-growth of tissue, protruding from carious exposure in lower molar. What may be the possible diagnosis?
    - **A. Pulp polyp**
    - B. Pulp hyperemia
    - C. Varicosed polyp
    - D. Pulpal granuloma

42. For checking the response EPT (electric pulp tester) use low current with high potential difference to stimulate
    A. A delta fibers
    B. A beta fibers
    C. C fibers
    D. B fibers

43. Electiveendodontictreatmentiscontraindicatedinpatientshavingmyocardialinfarctionwithinthepast6months,thisisbecause
    A. Local anaesthetic is absolutely contraindicated
    B. There is an increased susceptibility to infection
    C. There is an increased susceptibility of repeated infarctions
    D. Such patients should be treated in hospital under care of his physician

44. A10-year old child presents with mild discomfort in teeth #21 and #22. The teeth were traumatized the day before in a fall from a motorcycle. Clinical examination reveals both teeth are tender to percussion and the crowns are intact. Cold test using Endo-ice indicated that the teeth #21 and #22 are not responsive. Treatment plan for such case is
    A. Heat testing for teeth #21 and #22
    B. Partial pulpotomy for teeth #21 and #22
    C. Root canal treatment for teeth #21 and #22
    D. No treatment and follow-up of the patient over the next few weeks

45. Patients who present with dental pain which wakes them up at night would most likely be suffering from
    A. Chronic Periradicular Periodontitis
    B. Acute Traumatic periodontitis
    C. Reversible Pulpitis
    D. Irreversible Pulpitis

46. Patients are most likely to have associated sign of systemic infection when they present with
    - **A. Acute Periradicular Abscess**
    - B. Chronic Periradicular Abscess
    - C. Chronic Periradicular Periodontitis
    - D. Acute Traumatic Periodontitis

47. Which of the flowing is most likely to occur following the recent placement of an amalgam restoration with inadequate occlusal contour
    - A. Acute Periradicular abscess
    - B. Chronic Periradicular abscess
    - C. Chronic Periradicular periodontitis
    - **D. Acute traumatic periodontitis**

48. Which of the following is most often associated with a draining sinus
    - A. Acute Periradicular abscess
    - **B. Chronic Periradicular abscess**
    - C. Reversible pulpitis
    - D. Irreversible pulpitis

49. The failure of root canal treatment is most likely to result from
    - A. Apical leakage of the root canal filling
    - **B. Contamination of the pulp space with saliva**
    - C. Marginal leakage of the coronal restoration
    - D. Inadequate condensation of the root filling

50. The strongest evidence for a suspected root perforation in an endodontically treated tooth restored with a post retained crown is
    - A. Clinical history and crown appearance
    - B. Crown appearance and post not in line with root canal
    - **C. Clinical history and bone loss adjacent to post**
    - D. Root filling quality and post length

51. Mineral trioxide aggregate is a suitable repair material for perforation in tooth because.
    A. It is bio-compatible and forms a bacteria tight seal
    B. It forms a bacterial tight seal and has an aesthetic appearance
    C. It has an aesthetic appearance and is hard when set
    D. It is hard when set and is bactericidal

52. Peri-radicular surgery is indicated when
    A. A. The root canal filling does not reach the root apex and the tooth is tender to palpation
    B. B. The root canal filling is inadequately condensed and the tooth is mobile
    C. The root canal filling is satisfactory and the tooth is tender to palpation
    D. The root canal filling is too long and the tooth is asymptomatic

53. Mineral trioxide aggregate (MTA) is a useful root end filling material because
    A. It has a fast set and sets in the presence of moisture
    B. It is easy to place and sets slowly
    C. It is biocompatible and seals root end cavity well
    D. It bonds to dentine and is antibacterial

54. A 50-year-old male with a previous history of deep vein thrombosis (DVT), for which is he now takes warfarin, requests advice about analgesia following root canal therapy. Which of the following drugs would you advise?
    A. Aspirin formulation
    B. Ibuprofen formulation
    C. Diclofenac formulation
    D. Codeine-acetaminophen formulation

55. Intracanal medicament, Ledermix, is a combination of
    A. Ciprofloxacin, Minocycline, Metronidazole
    B. Triamcinolone acetonide, Demeclocycline
    C. Amoxycillin, Metronidazole
    D. Erythromycin, Gentamycin

56. Which of the following is not a main reason for using rubber dam during root canal treatment?
    A. Provides retraction of the soft tissues
    B. **Help manage an uncooperative patient.**
    C. Protects against the risk of inhalation or ingestion of endodontic instruments and irrigants
    D. Eliminates microbial contamination, via saliva, of the exposed root canal System

57. During history taking, a patient complains of pain. Which of the following characteristics of the pain complaint is least relevant?
    A. Character
    B. Severity
    C. Tolerance
    D. Radiation

58. From the list below, which is an unlikely characteristic of reversible pulpitis?
    A. Sharp transient pain
    B. Pain often poorly localized
    C. Pain lingers when stimulus removed
    D. No obvious radiographic changes

59. Which of the following is not a reason for failure to achieve adequate anaesthesia?
    A. Inadequate amounts of local anesthesia administered
    B. Resistance due to lack of inflammation
    C. Poor clinical technique
    D. Variation in patient's anatomy

60. The normal interstitial pulpal pressure is approximately
    A. 1-5mmHg
    B. 6-10mm Hg
    C. 13-15mm Hg
    D. 15-35mm Hg

61. The nerve fibres responsible for pulpal pain transmission
    A. A beta and C nerve fibres
    B. A beta and A delta nerve fibres
    C. A alpha and A delta nerve fibres
    D. A delta and C nerve fibres

62. Structure rich in proprioceptors
    A. Odontoblastic layer
    B. Stroma of dental pulp
    C. Periapical area
    D. Dentin layer

63. A 'hot tooth' is defined as that tooth
    A. Difficult to anesthetize
    B. With pink coronal discoloration
    C. With large red mass in the pulp chamber
    D. With hyperaemic pulp

64. A patient returns two days after routine composite restoration complaining of severe sharp pain to thermal changes particularly cold. Thermal testing shows sharp momentary response. Response to percussion and palpation test is with in normal limits. The ideal emergency treatment to relieve the patient's complaint is
    A. Check the marginal seal of the restoration and apply desensitizer
    B. Removal of restoration and temporization
    C. Endodontic access and pulp extirpation
    D. Anti-inflammatory and antibiotic prescription

65. Which among the following is more likely to undergo ‘flare up’ after single visit root canal treatment?
    A. Symptomatic irreversible pulpitis
    B. Asymptomatic irreversible pulpitis
    C. Asymptomatic apical periodontitis
    D. Chronic apical abscess

66. The pain from exposed dentin is due to
    A. Inflammatory mediators that stimulate nerve fibres
    B. Exposed nerve fibres at the DEJ
    C. Thermal changes that damage the C fibres
    D. Movement of fluids inside the dentinal tubules

67. Endodontic treatment is contraindicated when
    A. The canal appears to be calcified
    B. A large Periapical lesion is present
    C. **The patient has no motivation to maintain the tooth**
    D. The tooth needs periodontal crown lengthening before restoration

68. Single-visit root canal treatment is indicated in case of
    A. Necrotic pulps with apical abscess
    B. Symptomatic irreversible pulpitis with apical periodontitis
    C. Asymptomatic irreversible pulpitis with apical periodontitis
    D. Symptomatic irreversible pulpitis without any apical changes

69. In primary endodontics with secondary periodontal lesions, the treatment plan is
    A. Perio treatment only
    B. Endo treatment only
    C. Endo treatment followed by perio treatment
    D. Perio treatment followed by endo treatment

70. A 33-year-old female patient is suffering repeatedly from swelling in relation to her right central and lateral incisor. Clinically, deep palatal pockets with extensive attachment loss were detected related to the lingual aspect of the lateral incisor. The pulp test was positive and radiographically massive bone loss was evident along the whole root of the lateral incisor. The diagnosis is
    A. **Localized periodontal disease related to a developmental groove defect**
    B. Marginal periodontitis related to upper anterior teeth
    C. Chronic apical periodontitis related to necrosed lateral incisor
    D. Primary periodontal lesion with secondary endodontic involvement

71. Predisposing clinical condition for endodontics flare up is
    A. Acute periapical abscess
    B. Acute apical periodontitis
    C. **Asymptomatic necrotic pulp with periapical lesion**
    D. Pain and swelling since the treatment

72. **The most common cause of discoloration of non-vital teeth is**
    A. Fluorosis
    B. **Haemorrhage into the pulp chamber**
    C. By production of some illnesses
    D. Coffee

73. A 22 years old male patient came to your office early in the morning complaining of pain that awakened him at 2:00 AM last night and did not allow him to sleep till he came to your office, this patient most probably has
    A. Reversible pulpitis
    B. **Irreversible pulpitis**
    C. Trauma from occlusion
    D. Pulp polyp

74. 20-year-old male patient came with severe pain on biting related with upper first molar. On clinical examination, no caries, good oral hygiene, no changes in radiograph. Patient had history of fixed prosthesis 3 days back. What is the diagnosis?
    A. Pulp necrosis
    B. Acute apical periodontitis
    C. Chronic apical abscess
    D. Acute reversible pulpitis

75. All are characteristics of irreversible pulpitis *except*
    A. Dull, localized pain
    B. Duration is a few minutes to an hour
    C. Sometimes spontaneous pain with no external stimuli
    D. **Pain resolves with removal of stimulus**

76. Ideal root canal morphology is
    A. Conical
    B. Cylindrical
    C. **Three dimensional**
    D. Predictable

77. Pain on percussion before endodontic treatment suggests
    A. Reversible pulpitis
    B. Irreversible pulpitis
    C. Pulp necrosis
    D. **Inflammation of periodontal tissues**

78. A young, 12-year boy presents with reddish overgrowth of tissue, protruding from carious exposure in lower molar. What may be the possible diagnosis?
    A. Pulp polyp
    B. Pulp hyperemia
    C. Varicosed polyp
    D. Pulpal granuloma

79. To help prevent external transportation
    A. Precurve instruments
    B. Use large instruments
    C. Avoid use of Sodium hypochlorite
    D. Use vigorous instrument

80. Reversible pulpitis
    A. Severe inflammation of pulp tissue
    B. Yields a negative response to electric pulp testing
    C. **Yields a positive response to thermal pulp testing**
    D. Requires RCT

81. All are the features of irreversible pulpitis *except*
    A. pain by hot or cold stimuli, or pain that occurs spontaneously
    B. Pain is boring or gnawing severe pain
    C. Pain on bending or lying
    D. **Pain lasts for few seconds**

82. The crown-down preparation advocates beginning radicular access with
    A. A smaller instrument first
    B. Pre curvature of smaller instrument
    C. A larger instrument first
    D. Removal of the clinical crown

83. Which of the following is most likely to increase accuracy, negotiate curved canals and reduce force of instrumentation?
    A. Carbon steel file
    B. **NITI Instrument**
    C. Reamers
    D. H-file

84. Patient came with severe pain related to right mandibular 1st molar, there is no related swelling, pulp test is negative, no evidence on radiograph. What will be diagnosis?
    A. Irreversible pulpitis
    B. Acute periodontal abscess
    C. Suppurative abscess
    D. Acute pulpitis

85. Patient came to clinic, had a root canal treatment of mandibular first molar 2 years back, upon X-ray you found radiolucency with bone resorption in one root only, what will be your treatment plan
    A. Redo RCT
    B. Intracanal medicaments
    C. Root amputation
    D. Periodontal curettage

86. Root canal contraindicated in
    A. Vertical fracture of root
    B. Diabetic patient
    C. Unrestored tooth
    D. Periodontally involved tooth

87. Patient recalled to check the prognosis of the Root Canal treated tooth, will evaluate with
    A. To check the size of the lesion#
    B. No pain on percussion and palpation
    C. Presence of signs and symptoms
    D. Histological finding

88. Very small access opening in incisors leads to
    A. Complete removal of the pulp
    B. **Incomplete removal of pulp**
    C. Difficult in irrigation
    D. Conservative restoration

89. Irrigation solution for RCT that causes protein coagulation is
    A. Sodium Hypochlorite
    B. Iodine potassium
    C. **Formocresol**
    D. CHX

90. Male patient came to your clinic with continuous severe pain related to 1st maxillary molar. After examination dentist diagnose the tooth is carious and has irreversible pulpitis. He decides to do RCT. After enough time for anaesthetisation, the patient won't allow the dentist to touch the tooth due to severe pain. Dentist should
    A. Give another appointment to the patient with description of antibiotics
    B. Extraction
    C. Give intrapulpal anaesthia and continue the treatment
    D. Wait till anaesthsize the tooth

91. Patient with pain on the upper right area, and the patient cannot localize the tooth cause the pain, what is the least reliable way to do test pulp?
    A. Cold test
    B. Hot test
    C. Electric test
    D. Stimulation of the dentin

92. A 15-year-old male patient came with trauma on the central incisal a year ago, and have discolouring on it, in the exam, no vitality in this tooth, and in the x-ray there is fracture from the edge of the incisal to the pulp, and wide open apex the best treatment
    A. Apexification
    B. Apexogenesis
    C. RCT with gutta-percha
    D. Pulp capping

93. All of the following are contraindicated to Endodontic treatment *except*
    A. Non restorable tooth
    B. Vertical root fracture
    C. Tooth with insufficient bone support
    D. Patient has diabetes or hypertension

94. Patient returned to you after 1 month from doing amalgam restoration with definite severe pain, should do to all of the above *except*
    A. Check the tooth for supra occlusion
    B. Radiograph
    C. Re-restoration
    D. Endodontic treatment

95. The patient has dull pain and swelling and IOPA shows apical radiolucency, your diagnosis will be
    A. Acute periodontal abscess
    B. Phoenix abscess
    C. Chronic abscess
    D. Irreversible pulpitis

96. Initial thermal and electric pulp testing of traumatized teeth
    A. Establish the base line to physiological status of the pulp
    B. If positive, can be assumed to indicate healthy pulp
    C. If negative, means RCT should be done
    D. Should be repeated after 30 days to finalize the pulp condition

97. Which of the following is true regarding the apical foramen?
    A. The diameter remains constant throughout life
    B. The position of the apical foramen is often visible on radiograph
    C. **The foramen is most commonly located 0.5mm to 1.0mm away from the anatomic root apex**
    D. Unpredictable

98. Which of the following irrigant has the property of "Substantivity"?
    A. Sodium hypochlorite
    B. **Chlorhexidine gluconate**
    C. EDTA
    D. Normal saline

99. Intracanal medication is indicated for
    A. Canal obturation
    B. Canal cleaning and disinfection
    C. Drying the canal
    D. Preventing operative pain

100. Patient came with the pain and swelling after 1st appointment of root canal treatment, what will be the reason-
    A. Improper diagnosis for RCT
    B. Endodontic Flare up
    C. Medication
    D. Due to vital tooth RCT

References

Fouad, Ashraf F. *Endodontic Microbiology.* 1st edition; 2017. *Quintessence.* ISBN: 978-08-1382-646-2. ISBN: 978-16-0795-192-6.

Gopikrishna, V., Chandra, Subhash. *Grossman's Endodontic Practice.* 13th edition; 2014. Wolters Kluwer. ISBN: 978-81-8473-918-6.

Gutmann, James L., Lovdahl, Paul E. *Problem Solving in Endodontics.* 5th edition; 2011. Elsevier Mosby. ISBN: 978-03-2306-888-8.

Hargreaves, Kenneth M, *Cohen's Pathways of Pulp.* 1st South Asian edition; 2016. Elsevier. ISBN: 978-81-3124-304-6.

Kohli, Anil. *Text book of Endodontics.* 1st edition; 2009. Elsevier. ISBN:978-81-3122-181-5.

Merino, Enrique M.Endodontic Microsurgery. 1st edition; 2009. *Quintessence.* ISBN:978-18-5097-178-8.

Rotstein, Ilan, Ingle, John I. 7 th edition;2016. *PMPH-USA*. ISBN: 978-16-0795-192-6.

Shenoy, Arvind. Mala, Kundabala. *Endodontics-Principles & amp; Practice.* 1st edition; 2016. Elsevier. ISBN: 978-81-3124-448-7.

Torabinejad, Mahmoud, Walton, Richard E., Fouad, Ashraf F. *Endodontics-Principles & Practice.* 5th edition; 2014. Elsevier. ISBN: 978-14-5575-410-6.

In: Scenario Based MCQ in Dentistry ISBN: 978-1-53617-298-0
Editors: M. Khursheed Alam et al. © 2020 Nova Science Publishers, Inc.

Chapter 7

SCENARIO BASED MCQS IN ORTHODONTICS

Mohammad Khursheed Alam[1] ***and Ibadullah Kundi***[2]
[1]Orthodontics, HOD Preventive Dentistry Department,
College of Dentistry, Jouf University, Aljouf, Saudi Arabia
[2]Orthodontics, Preventive Dentistry Department, College of Dentistry,
Jouf University, Aljouf, Saudi Arabia

This chapter intended to cover scenario based MCQ from the discipline of orthodontics. The word orthodontic derived from two Greek words – 'Orthos' means right or correct and 'Dons' means tooth. The term orthodontics was internationally used by Frenchman, LeFoulon in 1839.The branch of dental science which deals with the normal growth and development of the body generally, jaws and teeth particularly; their variation and abnormalities and prevention and treatment of dentofacial abnormalities within accepted range of normal.

Orthodontics is a branch of Clinical Stomatology, the mechanisms of major research and development of dentofacial deformities, diagnosis, prevention and treatment. The area and specialty of dentistry concerned with the supervision, guidance and correction of the growing or mature dentofacial structures, including those conditions that require movement of teeth or correction of malrelationships and malformations of their related structures and the adjustment of relationships between and among teeth and facial bones by the application of forces and/or the stimulation and redirection of functional forces within the craniofacial complex. According to World Health Organization (WHO), malocclusion can be defined as "a dento-facial anomaly refers to irregular occlusion and/or abnormal craniofacial relationships, which may interrupt aesthetic appearance, function, facial harmony, and psychosocial well-being". Major responsibilities of orthodontic practice include the diagnosis, prevention, interception and treatment of all forms of malocclusion of the teeth and associated alterations of their surrounding structures; the design, application and control of functional and corrective appliances; and the guidance of the dentition and its supporting structures to attain and maintain optimal occlusal relations, physiologic function and esthetic harmony of facial and cranial structures. A malformation of the teeth, jaws and/or face characterized by disharmonies of size, form and/or function. The term encompasses problems such as malocclusion, cleft lip and palate and other skeletal or soft tissue anomalies, or syndromes that involve the face and the dentoalveolar complex. The manifestation of Dentofacial Deformity are: a. malposition of individual, abnormity of arch form, tooth malalignment, b. maxillomandibular malrelationship and c. malrelationship between jaw and cranium.

1. Mr. Ahmed came to dental clinic with the complaint that there is a Labial displacement of left & right maxillary canines in his son's mouth. On examination there was crowding in maxillary anterior segment due to lack of space. What can be the most possible reason?
   A. Eruption of maxillary canine before that of maxillary first premolar
   B. Eruption of maxillary lateral incisor before that of maxillary canine

C. Eruption of maxillary canine before that of maxillary lateral incisors
D. Eruption of maxillary first premolar before that of maxillary canine

2. A 16-year-old male patient is involved in chronic mouth breathing since childhood due to enlarged tonsils. During the clinical examination his facial profile will be?
   A. convex profile, short face
   B. concave profile, short face
   C. convex profile, long face
   D. concave profile, long face

3. An 8-year-old child came to the dental clinic for a routine examination. Which one of the following will not be considered by the Dentist while he examines the Gingiva of the patient?
   A. Contour
   B. Stippling
   C. sulcus depth
   D. depth of vestibule

4. Mr. Bilal came to dental clinic with is baby with a complaint that the baby has fever for the past 2 days and that the baby cries a lot. On examination there was a swelling in the posterior aspect of gingiva. Intra oral x-ray revealed that primary second molar was in erupting stage. What is the age of the baby patient?
   A. 8-14 months
   B. 14-20 months
   C. 20-30 months
   D. 30-36 months

5. A father brought his four sons for dental checkup. On examination all had class III skeletal pattern with constricted maxilla. But the father was explained that expansion will be more effective only in one of the children. The midpalatal suture is most likely to open at which of following ages of expansion?
    A. 33-year-old
    B. 13-year-old
    C. 43-year-old
    D. 23-year-old

6. A young 16-year-old male patient came to the dental clinic with a complaint of a loose fitting removable Hawley's retainer appliance which was given to him 1 months back by his orthodontist and was advised to get it activated every month. The new dentist will activate the appliance by compressing the
    A. Center of Base plate
    B. Bridge of Adam clasp
    C. U loop of Labial bow
    D. Arrow heads of Adam clasp

7. Hisham came for orthodontic consultation and gave history that he recently had a root canal treatment done for his left central incisor. Will it be possible for the orthodontist to do the orthodontic movement of that teeth?
    A. Yes
    B. No
    C. Maybe
    D. Poor prognosis

8. An 8-year-old female patient had multiple severely decayed deciduous teeth. As she had mixed dentition what will be the dentist's treatment protocol?
    A. Extraction of decayed teeth & space regaining
    B. Extraction of decayed teeth & space maintenance
    C. space maintenance without extraction of decayed teeth

D. space regaining without extraction of decayed teeth

9. Abdul a 20-year-old boy went to his dentist with a complaint of spacing between his upper central incisors. On examination there was presence of mid line diastema. There was a high frenal attachment. Which test will the dentist do to confirm it?
   A. Montoux test
   B. Cotton test
   C. Ganong's test
   D. Blanch test

10. Rehman's cephalometric Stiener's analysis values were as follows. Angle S.N.A = 86°, Angle S.N.B = 80°. What was the orthodontist's interpretation for the patient's skeletal pattern?
    A. Skeletal class I
    B. Skeletal class I
    C. Skeletal class I
    D. Skeletal class IV

11. Mohammed's molar relation was as follows: for both left & right side the upper 1st permanent molars mesio buccal cusp occluded posterior to the lower 1st permanent molars mesio buccal groove. What is the angle's molar classification?
    A. Angle class I molar relation
    B. Angle class II molar relation
    C. Angle class III molar relation
    D. Angle class II Div 1 molar relation

12. A child came to the dental clinic for checkup but was unable to tell his age? On intra oral examination there were presence of 12 erupted primary and 12 erupted permanent teeth. What is the age of the child?
    A. 6.5 years
    B. 8.5 years
    C. 11.5 years
    D. 13.5 years

13. Mr. Kareem brought his two children one female and one male for dental checkup. The female was 18-years-old & the male was 12 years old. Both had a skeletal class II growth pattern. The growth modification can be done only for the following
    - **A. Only in male**
    - B. Only in female
    - C. In both the male & female
    - D. Cannot be done

14. During Saudi licensing examination there was a question to the dental students that who is the "Father of modern orthodontics". What is the right answer?
    - A. Dr. Peirre Fauchard
    - B. Dr. P. R. Begg
    - C. Dr. E. H. Hartley
    - **D. Dr. E. H. Angle**

15. Alruwaily, a dental student was tracing Steiner's analysis on his patients cephalogram, the supervisor pointed at the A.N.B Angle and asked him what is it used to assess his right answer was?
    - A. Soft tissue profile
    - **B. Sagittal jaw discrepancy**
    - C. Crowding
    - D. Vertical jaw discrepancy

16. During an orthodontic clinical exam for the under graduate students patients study casts, photographs, opg & hand wrist radiograph was kept. The examiner asked which one of these is a supplemental diagnostic aid. What is the right answer?
    - **A. hand wrist radiographs**
    - B. OPG
    - C. Photographs
    - D. Study models

17. A rapid palatal expansion appliance was given to a patient with constricted maxilla. The patient asked what the rate of separation per day is. What was the dentists answer?
    A. 0.6 to 0.9 mm per day
    B. 0.4 to 0.7 mm per day
    C. 0.2 to 0.5 mm per day
    D. No movement per day

18. A radiologist opened a new radiographic clinic & invited his orthodontist friend to inaugurate his new x-ray machine. The orthodontist wanted to check the quality of the x ray film so he called his assistant to pose as patient. What should be the focal film distance for the lateral cephalogram?
    A. 2 feet
    B. 3 feet
    C. 4 feet
    D. 5 feet

19. A parent came to the dentist with a 1-month old child with a complaint that the child has erupted lower deciduous incisors since birth and it was difficult to milk feed the child. What is this type of teeth called as?
    A. Nonvital teeth
    B. Super latent teeth
    C. Neonatal teeth
    D. Pre grotal teeth

20. During an orthodontic exam, the examiner wrote 4 types of upper permanent teeth eruption sequence. Mostafa a dental student selected the right answer. What was it?
    A. 6-1-2-3-4-5-7
    B. 6-2-1-3-4-5-7
    C. 6-1-2-4-3-5-7
    D. 7-1-2-3-4-5-6

21. Malala a female patient of 26 years had a midline diastema and a high frenal attachment. The dentist advised her a surgical procedure during the fixed mecanotherapy. What is the name of that procedure?
    A. Circumferential osteotomy
    B. Pericoronotomy
    C. Frenectomy
    D. Apisectomy

22. A patient was advised a rapid palatal expansion appliance. He asked his orthodontist what will be the schedule of activation of that appliance. What did the orthodontist answer?
    A. Once weekly
    B. Twice weekly
    C. Twice daily
    D. Once monthly

23. The father of a 10-year-old girl is concerned about a 1.6 mm diastema between the child's upper central incisors. A very fibrous upper frenum is present and inserts on the palatine papilla. When tension is applied to the frenum, the papilla blanches. The management of choice is to
    A. Maxillary frenectomy to allow the teeth to close
    B. Close the space orthodontically
    C. Postpone treatment until complete eruption of upper canines
    D. Close the space with composite/veneer

24. Routine radiographic examination of a 7-year-old boy discloses supernumerary tooth between maxillary central incisors. The dentist should
    A. Delay removal of supernumerary tooth until its complete eruption
    B. Wait until the boy is 12 years of age to remove the supernumerary tooth

C. Remove the supernumerary tooth only if it develops a cyst.

D. Remove the supernumerary tooth as soon as possible without injury to the central incisors.

25. 13-year-old boy undergoing maxillary expansion, came to your clinic with his father. His father is a Dentist. Father was concerned about retention period for which the appliance is worn after completion of maxillary expansions. The retention period will be

A. 1 month

B. 3 months

C. 5 months

D. 9 months

26. A dentist mother was concerned about her daughter's orthodontic treatment. Her daughter has skeletal class II div. 1. She is 14 years old (early permanent dention). Which appliance is suitable for her case?

A. Herbst appliance

B. Twin block appliance

C. Either A or B

D. Fixed appliance

27. A dentist mother was concerned about her daughter's orthodontic treatment. Her daughter has skeletal class III. She is 8 years old. Which appliance is not suitable for such case?

A. Frankel III

B. Chincap

C. Reverse pull headgear

D. Maxillary splint appliance

28. Dentist father worried about his son. 8-year-old son having tongue thrusting. He is very much concerned. Tongue thrusting habit is often exaggerated by
    - **A. Enlarged tonsil**
    - B. Tongue-tie
    - C. Cross bite
    - D. Prognathic mandible

29. Routine Orthodontic history revealed that, the patient has thumb sucking habit. Prolonged thumb sucking directly results in all of the following *except*
    - **A. Deep over bite**
    - B. Proclination of upper central incisors
    - C. Rotation of upper laterals
    - D. Constriction of maxilla

30. 3rd year dental student was concerned about his malocclusion problem. He is worried to know the most common reason for malocclusion
    - A. Hypothyroidism
    - B. Presence of supernumerary teeth
    - **C. Early loss of primary teeth**
    - D. Late eruption of permanent teeth

31. A cardiologist father of a 9-year-old child concerned about his child's deep skeletal bite. Which of the following features can be seen in such case?
    - A. High mandibular plane
    - B. Deep palate
    - **C. Low mandibular plane**
    - D. All of the above

32. An orthodontic case management relates with the pubertal growth spurt. Which is the indicator of pubertal growth spurt?
    A. Sesamoid bone and hook of hamate
    B. Cervical vertebra
    C. Left lower canine
    D. All of the above

33. An intern dentist was concerned about pubertal growth spurt. When hand-wrist radiograph is not available what could be the other alternative to assess the pubertal growth spurt in your daily practice?
    A. Periapical intra-oral mandibular radiograph
    B. Orthopantomogram
    C. Cephalogram
    D. Bitewing films

34. 56-year-old patient with multiple missing of posterior teeth resulting in overclosure of the mandible. This can lead to
    A. Clicking of temporomandibular joint
    B. Destruction of the articular disc
    C. Crepitus
    D. None of the above

35. 19-year-old young lady complaints about long face. She feels that her face is longer than the normal. What is the ideal proportion of upper facial height to lower facial height?
    A. 45% : 55%
    B. 55% : 45%
    C. 50% : 50%
    D. 40% : 60%

36. Your brother always taking breath using mouth instead of nose. His face looks like adenoid faces (mouth breather). Facial profile of such condition characterized by
    A. Long and wide
    B. Long and narrow
    C. Short and wide
    D. Short and narrow

37. Your 5-year-old small brother has anteroposterior discrepancy in skeletal base. What is the best time to correct such problems?
    A. Mixed dentition period
    B. Primary dentition period
    C. Permanent dentition period
    D. Post-permanent dentition period

38. Malocclusion can be resulting from abnormal activity of orofacial muscle. The instrument most often used for evaluating the activity of orofacial muscles
    A. Holograph
    B. Bronchoscope
    C. Tonometer
    D. Electromyograph

39. 9-year-old patient with mixed dentition. In mixed dentition, which of the following may be considered as a self-correcting problem with age?
    A. Unilateral loss of primary canine
    B. Lack of interdental spaces
    C. A distal step
    D. Open bite

40. 24-Year-old male patient undergoing orthognathic surgery due to maxillary retrognathism. Most common choice of extraction in skeletal Class III due to maxillary deficiency, patient planned for orthognathic surgery is
    A. Maxillary 1st premolars only
    B. Mandibular 1st premolars only
    C. Maxillary 1st premolars and mandibular 2nd premolars
    D. Maxillary 2nd premolars and mandibular 1st premolars

41. During the treatment of a class II malocclusion, the anterior overjet is found to be increasing, this may be the result of
    A. Expansion of maxillary alveolar arch
    B. Loss of anchorage
    C. Loss of retention
    D. Unfavorable growth of the skull

42. An 11-year-old patient reported with gross skeletal discrepancy with ANB = + 8°, vertically high angle and incompetent lips. He was suggested to treat with
    A. Orthodontic camouflage
    B. Growth modification
    C. Orthognathic surgery
    D. Orthodontics & surgery

43. A 13-year-old girl presented with class II Div 1 malocclusion. Her Cephalometric analysis revealed a high angle tendency but with no Sagittal discrepancy. She was best treated with one of the following mechanics
    A. Bicuspid extractions
    B. Class II elastics
    C. Low pull HG
    D. Molar distalization

44. An 18-year-old working lady presented with severe sagittal maxillary excess and increased overjet. She was treated ultimately with one of the following surgical techniques?
    A. BSSO
    B. Maxillary advancement
    C. Maxillary impaction
    D. Wassmond procedure

45. A 12 years old boy with a class II div I presents for orthodontic treatment. There is a history of trauma involving tooth 8, which is asymptomatic. The following may happen during or after the conclusion of orthodontic treatment
    A. Bone resorption
    B. Loss of vitality
    C. Periapical infection
    D. Root resorption

46. What is the treatment of choice for a lingually erupted maxillary incisor in a 7-year-old with the rest of the occlusion normal?
    A. Inter-arch elastics
    B. No treatment
    C. Myo-functional appliance therapy
    D. Maxillary appliance applying labial force

47. An 8 years old patient presents with disto-occlusion. Cast and space analysis revealed an over jet of 4mm and discrepancy of 5mm, with a shift of lower midline towards right side. There was a history of premature loss of ‘c’. He was advised with one of the following treatment options on priority.
    A. Balancing extraction
    B. Compensatory extraction
    C. Molar distalization
    D. Serial extraction

48. A baby was born with severe respiratory embarrassment, short mandible and cleft palate, he was diagnosed with one of the following congenital anomaly
    A. Cleidocranial dysplasia
    B. Crouzon's syndrome
    C. Pierre Robin sequence
    D. Treacher Collin's syndrome

49. The Cephalometric evaluation of a 15-year-old female patient seeking orthodontic treatment shows increased palatal plane angle, a short ramus, short corpus length, high glenoid fossa relative to sella turcica, an obtuse gonial angle and a large anterior facial height. These characteristics are associated with
    A. Skeletal open bite
    B. Cross Bite
    C. Skeletal deep bite with class II malocclusion
    D. Skeletal open bite with class I malocclusion

50. A discrepancy of 7 mm was found in the mixed dentition analysis, the following management protocol will be required
    A. Space maintenance
    B. Space regaining
    C. Space supervision
    D. Serial extraction

51. A severe high angled case with short mandible in growing stage may be better treated with one of the following appliances
    A. Anderson appliance
    B. Activator
    C. Bionator
    D. Combined activator Headgear appliance

52. After Bolton analysis overall ratio showed value of more than 91.3, it will show
    A. Excessive mandibular tooth mass
    B. Excessive maxillary tooth mass
    C. Some macrodontia in the maxillary arch
    D. Some microdontia in the mandibular tooth mass

53. A 7 years old girl presents in early mixed dentition. On examination a functional unilateral cross bite is evident. The following is the right course of action
    A. Initiate a fixed appliance therapy
    B. Put in a quad helix
    C. Put the child on a high pull head gear
    D. Reassure the parent and put the child on a 6-month recall

54. A seven-year-old child with good occlusion has an in-standing lateral incisor (single tooth cross bite). There is sufficient room for alignment. What should be the best course of treatment?
    A. Correct the condition with a removable appliance
    B. Correct the condition with fixed appliance.
    C. Leave the tooth as it is
    D. Wait until the eruption of all permanent teeth.

55. A 9 years old girl is brought to your practice by her parents. You find out that the upper left lateral incisor is in cross-bite. The rest of the dentition looks normal and functional. You would
    A. Ask the lab technician to design an appropriate Upper RA.
    B. Plan a comprehensive fixed appliance treatment.
    C. Provide for disarticulation and a palatal spring in the prescription.
    D. Tell the parents that nothing needs to be done at this stage

56. In a class II div 1 case the extractions of the upper first premolars have been done. The fixed appliances were placed four months ago and the arches are completely aligned and leveled. The next step in the fixed orthodontic therapy would be
    A. Space closure
    B. Leveling
    C. Finishing
    D. Over-corrections

57. A severely rotated canine was derotated with fixed appliances in a 15yr old boy. How can the stability of the canine in its new position be increased?
    A. Supracrestal fibrotomy
    B. Papilla split incision
    C. Overcorrection of the derotation
    D. All of the above

58. Anchorage requirements of a patient with severe bimaxillary dento-alveolar protrusion and long face who is being treated with 1st premolar extractions can be termed as
    A. Maximum Anchorage
    B. Low Anchorage
    C. Moderate Anchorage
    D. Secondary Anchorage

59. In examining a 12-year-old boy, the dentist finds a deep anterior overlap, maxillary central incisors are lingually inclined, and maxillary lateral incisors protruded. Maxillary molars are in an anterior relationship with mandibular molars. The patient is likely to be
    A. Class I
    B. Class II Div I
    C. Class II Div II
    D. Supra class I

60. A worried mother comes to you with her 12-year-old son. She complains that the boy often gets ulceration of the gums behind the upper front teeth. After clinical examination and evaluation of diagnostic records it is revealed that she has a traumatic bite with an increased facial height. The treatment of choice to correct the deep bite would be
    A. High pull headgear
    B. Low pull headgear
    C. Anterior bite plane
    D. Utility archwires

61. An 11-year-old girl comes to you with a class II Div 2 skeletal malocclusion, and you have decided to correct the malocclusion with a functional appliance. The first line of action would be
    A. Install the functional appliance right away
    B. Give an anterior bite plane first
    C. Fixed appliance therapy followed by functional appliance insertion
    D. High pull headgear with a functional appliance.

62. A 10 year of age female reports with an isolated cross-bite of a permanent maxillary incisor in the mixed dentition. This problem is most often associated with
    A. An abnormal labial frenum
    B. Prolonged retention of a primary tooth
    C. Tongue thrusting
    D. Skeletal growth problem

63. You are going to perform cephalometric analysis of a patient, if the position of nasion is at fault, this will also influence ANB. The Eastman correction will be required to overcome this. This correction for ANB can only be applied for changes in the position of nasion, which of the following measurement will you consider to confirm that there is problem with the position of the nasion and not the Sella?

A. SN-MP angle
B. SN-PP angle
C. Interincisal angle
D. PP-MPangle

64. A patient with Cleidocranial dysplasia was treated with extraction of all primary and supernumerary teeth, and open surgical exposure of the permanent teeth, all carried out as one procedure, followed by direct orthodontic traction is carried out for treatment of impacted teeth. What do you think which one of the following approach was this?
A. Belfast Hamburg approach
B. Jerusalem approach
C. Open surgical exposure approach
D. Toronto Melbourne approach

65. Disturbances in initiation and proliferation stage of dental development may lead to one of the following anomalies
A. Anodontia and Oligodontia
B. Regional Odontodysplasia
C. Microdontia
D. Peg shaped teeth

66. A 40-year-old female is being treated for Class I crowding. She has been taking a drug for hyper calcemia. She has retarded tooth movement with braces. Which is the most likely drug she is taking?
A. ACE inhibitors
B. Anticonvulsant Phenytoin
C. Anti-malarial
D. Bisphosphonates

67. A patient with some missing permanent teeth, retained deciduous teeth and a few superneumarary teeth. Which of the following syndromes has the above clinical features?
    A. Aperts syndrome
    B. Cleiodocranial dysplasia
    C. Ectodermal dysplasia
    D. Gorlin Goltz syndrome

68. A patient with dentinogenesis imperfecta having shell teeth, with lose enamel and have poorly mineralized dentine leading to multiple pulp exposures. Which of the following type of dentine defect is this?
    A. Dentine dysplasia type I
    B. Dentine dysplasia type II
    C. Dentinogenesis imperfecta Type II
    D. Dentinogenesis imperfecta Type III

69. A patient presented with clinical features of down slanting palpabral fissures, zygomatic supraorbital and mandibuar hypoplasia, severe malformation of the ears, isolated cleft palate and Class II skeletal pattern with increased vertical proportion. The aetiology is neuro-cristopathy. Which of the following syndromes will have these clinical features?
    A. Apert syndrome
    B. Cleido-cranial dysplasia
    C. Crouzon's syndrome
    D. Mandibulo-facial dysostosis

70. One of the following cytokines is released during bone resorption process and helps stimulate subsequent bone formation
    A. Inter leukin B 1
    B. Osteo protegrin (OPG)
    C. Transforming growth factor Beta
    D. RANK

71. An orthodontist when installing head gear, rapid palatal expander or functional appliances utilizes one of the following process as dominant process to induce facial growth
    - A. Displacement
    - B. Drift
    - C. Mini modelling
    - **D. Modelling**

72. You are looking at the Orthopentotomogram of a patient, which of the following process cannot be seen on radiographs and can only be seen at the tissue level?
    - A. Cortical drift
    - **B. True Remodeling**
    - C. Deposition
    - D. Modelling

73. A 20-year-old female patient was treated with mandibular first premolar extractions. To increase the moment in the posterior segment you will prefer one of the following mechanics
    - A. Banding mandibular second molars
    - B. Buccal crown torque of posterior teeth
    - **C. Tip back bends**
    - D. Gable bends between first and second premolars

74. In an adult patient, at what point you will place the centre of rotation by changing the couple to force ratio to move it bodily?
    - A. At infinity
    - B. At the incisal edge
    - C. At the root apex
    - **D. Between centre of rotation and Apex**

75. A male patient 15-year-old presented with the family history of a malocclusion. The most probable malocclusion will be
    A. Mandibular asymmetry
    B. Maxillary asymmetry
    C. Narrow maxilla
    D. Prognathic mandible

76. A Class III malocclusion patient with one of the following readings according to discriminant analysis may not be treated by camouflage
    A. ANB6 degrees
    B. AO – BO distance -5 mm
    C. Lower incisors to mandibular plane angle of 95 degrees
    D. Wits -3 mm

77. Prospective research has failed to demonstrate one of the following findings about Self Ligating brackets
    A. Deleterious effects on periodontal ligament
    B. Decrease overall treatment duration and fewer deleterious effects of fixed appliances
    C. Reduce plaque accumulation
    D. Reduction in chair side assistance

78. In a growing adolescent when bone scan Te bisphosphonate a marker of bone activity, is performed. One of the following structure has high remodeling rate. What do you think which one is it?
    A. Alveolar process
    B. Basilar process
    C. Scapula
    D. Zygomatic bone of maxilla

79. A 40-year-old woman has decreased rate of tooth movement with the braces. This could be due to one of the following causes
    A. Decrease in the Estrogen level
    B. Decrease in Parathyroid level

C. Increase in Estrogen level
D. Hypercalcemia

80. In a severe class II division 1 malocclusion we would expect to find
    A. ANB angle of +80
    B. ANB angle of -80
    C. An ANB of +20
    D. ANB of 0

81. In a growing child, who is 8 years old, the periosteal bone growth associated with muscle function occurs at
    A. Capsular matrix
    B. Growth centre
    C. Growth site
    D. Primary growth site

82. A 9 years old girl is brought to your practice by her parents. You find out that the upper left lateral incisor is in crossbite. The rest of the dentition looks normal and functional. What will be your most appropriate treatment approach?
    A. Install a twin block.
    B. Plan a comprehensive fixed appliance treatment.
    C. Prescribe an upper Removable appliance with a finger spring.
    D. Provide for disarticulation and a palatal spring in the prescription

83. A patient 14 years old presented with supernumerary teeth, sclerotic bone and heavy fibrous gingival, crowding, early extraction of tooth germ. Which one of the following will be a potential complication due to these risk factors?
    A. Ectopic eruption
    B. Interference with eruption
    C. Transposition
    D. Traumatic displacement of teeth

84. While trying to locate a permanent canine in the upper arch, you decide to go for tube shift technique. When you moved the tube towards the right in horizontal plane, the canine appeared to have moved towards the left of the neighbouring teeth on the film, indicates that
    - **A. Canine is buccally placed**
    - B. Canine is near to the midline
    - C. Canine is right in the middle of the alveolus
    - D. Canine is palatally placed

85. During the development of craniofacial region, the upper lip philtrum, primary palate and central portion of the nose develops by the fusion of the following process
    - A. Two lateral nasal processes
    - B. Two Maxillary processes
    - C. Two Mandibular processes
    - **D. Two medial nasal processes**

86. 20 years old patient with the clinical features of hypoplasia of midface, craniosynostosis and syndactyly. What do you think which syndrome the patients are suffering from?
    - **A. Apert's syndrome**
    - B. Crouzon syndrome
    - C. Digeorge anomaly
    - D. Down's syndrome

87. A patient with clinical features of lower lip pitting and cleft lip and cleft palate, hypodontia and webbing of the soft tissues. Which one of the following will be your likely diagnosis?
    - A. Aperts syndrome
    - B. Cleiodocranial dysplasia
    - C. Treacher Collin's syndrome
    - **D. vander Woude syndrome**

88. In a 9-year-old child postnatal development of the nasomaxillary complex occurs via intramenbranous ossification with the exception of one of the following structures
    A. Alae of the none
    B. Alveolar arch
    C. Nasal septum
    D. Pterygoid plates

89. A 14 years old female patient presented to orthodontic clinic with a complaint of missing tooth in lower right quadrant. On examination her all permanent teeth were erupted till second molars except lower right second premolar. The right lower first molar was tilted mesially with inadequate space left for second premolar with fully formed crown and ¾ root development with no other pathology. What is your management protocol?
    A. Observe for next six months
    B. Remove the dentigerous cyst
    C. Soft tissue incision to allow eruption
    D. Orthodontics space opening

90. The second permanent molar is located in the ramus of the mandible of a 6 years old child. The same molar is located in the body of the mandible when the child reaches 13 years of age. The body of the mandible increases in length to accommodate the second molar by
    A. Apposition of bone in the in the condyle and cornoid processes
    B. Apposition of bone on the alveolar margins and lower surface of the body of mandible
    C. Apposition of bone at the symphysis and posterior surface of ramus of the mandible
    D. Resorption of bone along the anterior surface and deposition on the posterior surface of ramus

91. An 8 years old patient with flush terminal plane relationship and normal skeletal growth pattern presented with lower dental midline shifted towards right. Cast and space analysis revealed an over jet of 4 mm and arch length discrepancy of 5 mm. There was a history of premature loss of lower right "e". What treatment option will you advise on priority?
    A. Balancing extraction
    B. Compensatory extraction
    C. Molar distalization
    D. Serial extraction

92. The Cephalometric evaluation of a 15-year-old female patient seeking orthodontic treatment shows increased palatal plane angle, a short ramus, short corpus length, high glenoid fossa relative to sella turcica, an obtuse gonial angle and a large anterior facial height. These characteristics are associated with
    A. Skeletal open bite
    B. Skeletal deep bite
    C. Skeletal deep bite with class II malocclusion
    D. Skeletal open bite with class I malocclusion

93. A 13-year-old presented with bilateral posterior cross bite with constricted maxilla. His lower jaw is clock-wise rotated. The orthodontist gave RME and after expansion incorporated one of the following mechanics in follow up fixed orthodontics
    A. Buccal crown torque
    B. Buccal root torque
    C. Cross elastics
    D. Lingual crown torque

94. A 12 years old boy with a class II div I presents for orthodontic treatment. There is a history of trauma involving tooth 8, which is asymptomatic. The following may happen during or after the conclusion of orthodontic treatment

A. Loss of vitality
B. Periapical infection
C. Root resorption
D. Tooth discoloration

95. An OPG of 11 years old boy shows no signs of the third molar. This may imply the following
    A. Boys usually do not have third molars.
    B. May develop at a later stage
    C. OPG is not a diagnostic x-ray for third molar visualization at age 11.
    D. Third molars have been extracted

96. Features of epicanthal folds, flat nasal bridge, congenital heart defects, underdeveloped maxilla and disturbed number, timing and sequence of eruption correlate with
    A. Cleido-cranial dysplasia
    B. Cruzon's Syndrome
    C. Mandibulofacial synostosis
    D. Trisomy 21

97. A 5-year-old patient has gap vertically between her upper and lower teeth. Which one of the following could be the etiological factor?
    A. Clock wise rotation of the jaw
    B. Deep curve of Spee
    C. Thumb sucking
    D. Nail biting

98. A 12-year-old boy was given high pull Headgear. What could be the indication of using this orthopedic appliance?
    A. Deep bites
    B. Maxillary retrognathism
    C. Molar extrusion
    D. Molar intrusion

99. A 10-year-old patient has narrow maxilla and crowding in her front teeth. Palatal expansion is acquired by which one of the following appliances?
    A. Jasper jumper
    B. Herbst
    C. Quad helix
    D. Twin force

100. An orthodontic force is applied to a tooth of 19-year-old patient. How does alveolar bone respond to this orthodontic forces?
    A. Alveolar bone does not respond to orthodontic forces
    B. Alveolar bone is deposited in areas of tension and resorbed in area of pressure
    C. Alveolar bone expands in response to orthodontic forces
    D. Alveolar bone is resorbed in areas of tension and deposited in areas of pressure

References

Bhalajhi, SI. Orthodontics – *The art and science*. 4th edition., 2009.

Graber, TM; Vanarsdall, RL. *Orthodontics, Current Principles and Techniques, Diagnosis and Treatment Planning in Orthodontics*, D. M. Sarver, W.R. Proffit, J. L. Ackerman, Mosby, 2000.

Gurkeerat, Singh. *Textbook of Orthodontics*. 2nd edition. *Jaypee*, 2007.

Houston, S; Tulley. *Textbook of Orthodontics*. 2nd Edition. Wright, 1992.

Laura, M. *An introduction to Orthodontics*. 2nd edition. Oxford University Press, 2001.

Martyn, Cobourne; Andrew, Di Biase. *Handbook of Orthodontics*. Elsevier Health Sciences, 2015. ISBN: 9780723438076.

McNamara, JA; Brudon, WI. *Orthodontics and Dentofacial Orthopedics*. 1st edition, Needham Press, Ann Arbor, MI, USA, 2001.

Mitchel, L. *An Introduction to Orthodontics*. 3 editions. Oxford University Press., 2007.

Mohammad, EH. *Essentials of Orthodontics for dental students*. 3rd edition, 2002.

Mohammad, Khursheed Alam; Irfan, Qamruddin; Kathiravan, Purmal. *Malocclusion: Causes, Complications and Treatment*. Nova Science Publishers, NY, USA 2018. ISBN: 978-1-53613-123-9.

Proffit, WR; Fields, HW; Sarver, DM. *Contemporary Orthodontics*. 4th edition, Mosby Inc., St.Louis, MO, Elsevier. USA, 2012, ISBN: 978-0-323083171.

Samir, E. Bishara. *Textbook of Orthodontics*. Saunders 978-0721682891, 2002.

Sarver, DM; Proffit, WR. In TM Graber et al., eds., *Orthodontics: Current Principles and Techniques*, 4th ed., St. Louis: Elsevier Mosby, 2005.

Thomas, M. Graber; Katherine, WL. Vig; Robert, L. Vanarsdall. Jr. *Orthodontics: Current Principles and Techniques*. Mosby 9780323026215, 2005.

William, R. Proffit; Raymond, P. White; David, M. Sarver. *Contemporary treatment of dentofacial deformity*. Mosby 978-0323016971, 2002.

In: Scenario Based MCQ in Dentistry ISBN: 978-1-53617-298-0
Editors: M. Khursheed Alam et al.

Chapter 8

SCENARIO BASED MCQS IN PROSTHODONTICS

Mohammed G. Sghaireen, MDSc, Vinod Bandela, MDS, Saif Faruqi, MDS, Merin Mathew, PhD and Shital Sonune, MDS
Prosthodontics Department, College of Dentistry,
Jouf University, Aljouf, Saudi Arabia

Prosthodontics is one of the branches of dentistry that deals with the replacement of missing teeth and the associated soft and hard tissues by prostheses (crowns, bridges, dentures) which may be fixed or removable, or may be supported and retained by implants.

Prosthodontics is a broad specialty and the subspecialties are:

Fixed Prosthodontics: deals with restoration of teeth using crowns, bridges, onlays, inlays and veneers. All of the above-mentioned restorations are made in the dental laboratory on an impression of the mouth made by the Prosthodontist.

Removable Prosthodontics: Removable prosthodontics is concerned with prosthesis which replace the soft tissues and teeth and are more commonly referred to as dentures. These can be replacing all of the missing teeth (Complete dentures) or may be replacing some of the teeth (Partial dentures). Both of them can be replacing either the upper or lower arch or both. They can be solely made of plastic (acrylic) or can be made of a combination of metal and plastic. Fabrication of these prosthesis can take up to six visits or more and involves both clinic and laboratory steps.

Maxillofacial Prosthodontics: concerned with the rehabilitation of patients with congenital or acquired defects in the mouth or face. Congenital defects usually relate to cleft lip and palate. Acquired defects usually are due to cancer of the mouth or face and due to neurological defects, such as stroke. The prosthesis fabricated tends to fill up these defects. They are typically in the mouth and may include prosthesis such as Obturators, Speech bulbs, Palatal lifts, Palatal augmentation device to name a few; however, this branch also includes facial prosthesis like eye, ear, nose, facial, and other body parts like fingers, hands etc.

Maxillofacial prosthodontists are highly skilled prosthodontist who have advanced training in complex oral rehabilitation. They carry these treatments in a multi-disciplinary team usually consisting of maxillofacial surgeons, ENT surgeons, Plastic surgeons, neurosurgeons, speech and language pathologists and Clinical Oncologists. The overarching principle is to improve the quality of life of patients.

Implant Prosthodontics: A dental implant is an artificial device usually made of titanium or titanium alloys. It is a substitute for the root of a tooth and is generally shaped as a screw or cylinder. A successful implant provides a stable and rigid structure for retention or support of a bridge, denture or a maxillofacial prosthesis.

Properly placed implants have a high success rate and have high patient satisfaction with their use. They have to be placed with dentists who have acquired further competencies. The planning process for placement of implants is highly crucial and needs to be comprehensive for a successful outcome.

1. A 70 years old attended your office for replacement of his missing teeth. On intraoral examination, completely edentulous maxillary and mandibular arches. In making a final impression in this case, the most important area of the impression is
   A. Ridge area of maxilla and buccal shelf of mandible
   B. Lingual border area of the mandible
   C. Junction of hard and soft plate of maxilla and distolingual area of mandible
   D. Midpalatal area of maxilla and ridge of the mandible

2. A denture wearer patient attended your office complaining of unstable lower denture. On intraoral examination, peripheral seal seems to be fine. If you are making a new lower denture how can you enhance the stability?
   A. The level of occlusal plane is above the dorsum of the tongue
   B. The tongue rest on the occlusal surface of the lower teeth
   C. The lingual contour of the denture is concave
   D. The posterior teeth on the denture have a broad buccolingual width

3. When fabricating a complete denture the dentist should consider freeway space during jaw relations. Freeway space is defined as
   A. Vertical dimension at rest- vertical dimension of occlusion
   B. Vertical dimension of occlusion + vertical dimension at rest
   C. Vertical dimension at rest
   D. Vertical dimension at occlusion – vertical dimension at rest

4. A 50 years old patient complains of generalized sensitivity. upon examination, there was generalized attrition of the teeth, in this case the best way to locate hinge axis is
   A. Ear rods face-bow
   B. Maxillomandibular relations
   C. Kinematic face-bow
   D. Arbitrary face-bow

5. In complete denture patient Gothic arch tracer is a device used to record the following
    - A. Intraoral tracing device
    - B. Extraoral tracing device
    - **C. Centric relation and the movements of mandible in horizontal plane**
    - D. Records centric occlusion and the movements of mandible in vertical plane

6. During jaw relation in a complete denture patient, the first step in an arbitrary face-bow registration would be
    - A. Physiologic rest position
    - B. Inclination of each condyle
    - **C. Hing axis location**
    - D. Kinematic axis of movement of condyle

7. A diabetic patient with few remaining teeth attended your office. Upon examination you decided total extraction as the remaining teeth are hopeless. When categorizing the articulator, Bennett angle is related to
    - A. Condylar rotation
    - **B. Lateral bodily movement of mandible**
    - C. Protrusive movement of mandible
    - D. Edge to edge occlusion

8. A complete denture came back after 1 day of delivery complaining of clicking of denture during speaking. This is due to
    - **A. Increased vertical dimension of occlusion**
    - B. Increased interocclusal space
    - C. Decreased vertical dimension of occlusion
    - D. Using acrylic teeth against porcelain teeth

9. In a complete denture patient a semi-adjustable articulator was used. For obtaining lateral condylar guidance angle what formula the dentist should apply?
    A. L = 12 + D/H
    B. L = H/8 + 12
    C. L = H + 8/12
    D. L = H + D/12

10. A patient is complaining of soreness of the ridge few days after a denture delivery and elective grinding has been decided. This is best accomplished when the dentures are
    A. Rearticulated using original jaw relation record
    B. Rearticulated with a new series of jaw relation
    C. Equilibrated in the patients mouth
    D. Spot ground in the patient mouth

11. During jaw relation for a complete denture patient Willis gauge is used to measure
    A. Vertical height
    B. Bi-zygomatic width
    C. Interocclusal distance
    D. Interpupillary width

12. A medical-supply company shipped a semi-adjustable articulator to you. How could you make sure that this articulator is an Arcon one?
    A. The condylar heads are placed on the upper member of the articulator
    B. The condylar heads are placed on the lower member of the articulator
    C. The condylar elements are non-movable
    D. The inclination of condylar path is in a curved plane

13. A denture wearer patient came with some space between the denture and tissue of upper denture. When making reline impression the most common error would be
    - A. Failure to remove undercuts
    - B. Improperly rounded peripheries
    - C. Improper establishment of a post dam area
    - **D. Changed centric occlusion**

14. A male patient has visited the dental clinic complaining of redness over the denture bearing area. Upon examination a tissue conditioner has been seen on the fitting surface of the denture. The best explanation for this would be
    - A. a tissue conditioner can cause ridge resorption
    - **B. a tissue conditioner may harden in mouth**
    - C. a tissue conditioner is difficult to fabricate
    - D. a tissue conditioner is very irritant

15. Patient of high esthetic expectation came to the department of Prosthodontics for replacement of few missing teeth. The prosthodontist planned for immediate denture. But, one of the major disadvantage to immediate denture treatment is
    - A. The pain associated with the treatment
    - B. Difficulty in managing occlusions
    - **C. Need for reline**
    - D. No control over tooth placement and shape

16. A patient was planned an overdenture. The following are advantages of an overdenture *except*
    - A. Preservation of alveolar bone
    - **B. Aesthetically superior**
    - C. Enhanced Retention
    - D. Good

17. A young patient visited the college of Dentistry for replacement of his lower left posterior teeth. On examination there was missing 1st and 2nd molar. The prosthodontist planned for an implant supported fixed partial denture. The best bone for implant success is
    A. Spongy bone
    B. Cortical bone
    C. Lamellar bone
    D. Woven bone

18. Structural durability is considered to be one of the principles of teeth preparation to be crowned, this phenomenon is considered
    A. Biological phenomenon
    B. Mechanical phenomenon
    C. Structural phenomenon
    D. Physiological phenomenon

19. While preparing heavily restored mandibular right first molar, you find that the clinical crown height is less than 4 mm. As the patient has to travel back to his country in couple of days he did not have time for any crown lengthening procedure. So, as a prosthodontist, how can you obtain extra retention in this abutment tooth?
    A. Dovetail
    B. Slots, pins and grooves
    C. Outline form
    D. Decreasing tooth reduction

20. During diagnosis and treatment planning for a FPD Ante's law should be respected. In your opinion, if you want to apply this law while planning for fixed partial denture restoration it will provide an aid for
    A. Selection of pontic
    B. Selection of connector
    C. Selection of retainer
    D. Selection of abutments

21. The mechanical principle of tooth preparation plays a major role in overall success of the fixed partial denture prosthesis. You can obtain extra retention by different methods while preparing the tooth. Grooves are one of the features for enhancing retention. When you prepare grooves in vertical walls of bulk tooth structure it must be
    A. At least 1.0 mm
    B. At least 2.0 mm
    C. At least 1.5 mm
    D. At least 1.2 mm

22. A 45 years old patient came to your clinic asking for a restoration for his teeth. After clinical and radiographic examination, you found that the maxillary right first molar is endodontically treated with large restoration. You planned to make complete metal cast crown for this patient. What is the best choice for the finish line in this case?
    A. Chamfer
    B. Chamfer with bevel
    C. Feather edge
    D. Shoulder

23. A 50 years old patient demands for a gold crown for his teeth. Which type of gold alloy will you ask your technician to use to fabricate fixed partial denture?
    A. Soft gold
    B. Hard gold
    C. Medium gold
    D. Extra hard gold

24. A middle age patient visited you with the chief complaint of fracture of his tooth after root canal treatment. On examination, lingual cusp of his mandibular first molar tooth has chipped off. What is the best retainer of your choice in this case?
    A. Full veneer crown
    B. Partial veneer crown

C. 3/4 crown
D. 7/8 crown

25. In your fixed prosthodontic pre-clinical lab session, you were asked to do metal ceramic preparation for maxillary second premolar. How much occlusal reduction you will do for metal ceramic facing on the non-functional cusp?
    A. 0.5 – 1 mm
    B. 1 – 1.5 mm
    C. 1.5 – 2 mm
    D. 2 – 2.5 mm

26. After few days of cementation of metal ceramic crown, one of your patient came back with the complaint of fracture of ceramic covering. Which of the following laboratory technique should be used for stronger bonding of Porcelain to metal?
    A. Air firing
    B. Under compression
    C. Tempered after firing
    D. Several times firing before completion

27. In your fixed prosthodontic pre-clinical lab session, you were asked to do metal ceramic preparation for mandibular second molar. As per your knowledge, how much amount of occlusal reduction is required for functional cusp in metal-ceramic crown restoration?
    A. 1.0 – 2.5 mm
    B. 2.0 – 2.25 mm
    C. 1.5 – 2.0 mm
    D. 2.25 – 3 mm

28. A young athlete patient reported to the dental clinic with the complaint of repeated fracture of his 4-unit fixed partial denture. On examination it was found that the bridge cemented on his lower right posterior region was soldered in connector region. To avoid fracture in this

region the height of Connector for ceramic fixed partial denture should be

A. 2 mm
B. **4 mm**
C. 6 mm
D. 8 mm

29. As a dental graduate student, you were taught to understand the dental technician work and so you were taken to Dental laboratory. The technician told the students that in metal ceramic restoration, for greatest retention of the porcelain veneer, they are making the coping design as

A. Convex with undercuts
B. Concave with under
C. Convex with sharp angle
D. Convex with no undercut

30. Among the several patients who asked you for porcelain laminate veneers, which one is the most favorable for the veneers?

A. Teeth in parafunction
B. Heavily restored teeth
C. Closure of 1 mm diastema
D. Lower anterior teeth

31. The technician applies a layer of die spacer on the die to create a space for the luting agent, the ideal dimension for this luting agent space is

A. 0 – 20 microns
B. **20 – 40 microns**
C. 40 – 80 microns
D. 80 – 100 microns

32. A fixed partial denture is indicated to replace maxillary first and second premolars. The abutment teeth which are in normal alignment are canines and first molar. The connector of choice is
    A. Precision attachment on both canines and the molars
    B. A soldered joined on canines and a non-precision dovetail key way on the molar
    C. Soldered joint on the molar with submucosal rest on the canine
    D. Soldered joint on both canine and the molar

33. While fabricating the metal framework of a long span bridge the dental technician cast the framework in units and soldered the pieces together to form a single framework. To be biologically and mechanically acceptable, a soldered joint of a fixed bridge should be so formed that it
    A. Extend to the buccal margin of the retainer
    B. Extend the entire interproximal space occlusogingivally
    C. Thin occlusogingivally and thick buccolingually
    D. Depend on clasping and indirect retention

34. A patient came for post and core restoration on upper central incisor in which root canal treatment has been done, upon examination of the tooth before starting the treatment, the tooth was painful on percussion, the ideal treatment is
    A. To proceed with post and core restoration
    B. To give patient antibiotic and analgesics and proceed the post and core restoration
    C. To proceed post and core but don't make full crown until the tooth get relieve
    D. Don't make post and core

35. After the examination and diagnosis of the patient's clinical condition, it was decided to fabricate an upper complete denture and a mandibular implant supported complete denture. The minimum number of

implants required in mandible for the construction of the denture is usually

A. 2

B. 4

C. 6

D. 8

36. After the examination and diagnosis, the patient's partially edentulous state was classified as Kennedy's Class 1 and it was decided to fabricate a removable partial denture for the patient. The partial denture in this condition would receive its support

A. From the terminal abutments

B. Equally from abutment and the residual ridges

C. Mostly from residual ridge

D. Exclusively from residual ridge

37. Patient with recently delivered removable partial denture came to your clinic suffering from looseness of the denture. The main cause is

A. Deflective occlusal contact

B. Passive clasp on abutment

C. Thin flange

D. Insufficient overlap on posterior teeth

38. In examining aged patient wearing complete maxillary denture against six mandibular teeth, the clinician will see

A. Cystic degeneration of the foramina of the anterior palatine nerve

B. Loss of osseous structure in the anterior maxilla

C. Flabby tissue in the posterior region

D. Decrease interocclusal distance

39. 3 weeks after insertion of distal extension partial denture, the patient reported to the dental clinic with complaint of sensitivity to the chewing pressure. The most probable reason would be

A. Improper occlusion

B. Abrasion of tooth by clasp
C. Wearing off the cement base
D. Passive retentive arm

40. Many clinical situations such as distal extension partially edentulous conditions, require making functional impression of the arch, In a functional impression for RPD
    A. Teeth are recorded in anatomical form and ridge in functional form
    B. Teeth are recorded in functional form and ridge in anatomical form
    C. Teeth and ridge are recorded both in anatomical and functional form
    D. None of above

41. A composite restoration was done on a patient who preferred aesthetic restoration. During finishing, small air voids appear on the surface of the self-cured composite restoration. What may be the causative factor for small air voids appearance on the surface during finishing?
    A. Use of lubricants on the insertion instrument
    B. Insertion of material by incremental technique
    C. Dispensed composite exposed to operatory light before incremental insertion
    D. No lubricants on insertion instrument

42. A patient approached the dental clinic complaining the marginal discoloration of the composite restoration done one year back. Which of the following may be the factor that does not contribute for the bond failure of a one year old composite restoration with penetrating marginal discoloration?
    A. residual stress from polymerization shrinkage
    B. contamination at the margins during material insertion
    C. fatigue stress due to thermal cycling
    D. Insertion of material by incremental technique

43. The enamel portion of the tooth was etched with phosphoric acid for 15 seconds. Upon observation the tooth does not appear frosty. What may be the reason?
    - **A. Tooth may contain high fluoride level than normal**
    - B. Phosphoric acid is not ideal for etching enamel
    - C. Etching should have been done with phosphoric acid for 10 seconds
    - D. Etching should have been done with phosphoric acid for5 minutes

44. High strength Die material was used to pour an elastomeric impression, while removing from impression, the cast fractured. How it could be avoided?
    - A. by removing the die during its initial setting period
    - **B. vacuum mixing of die material to ensure less porosity**
    - C. by increasing the water to powder ratio than recommended
    - D. Increase the water temperature to boiling for mixing

45. A 50 year old male patient came to the clinic for partial denture treatment. The primary impression was made using alginate material. The impression appeared grainy with poor surface details. What may be the reason for it?
    - **A. Hot water used for mixing**
    - B. Vigorous figure -8- spatulation was done
    - C. During mixing, the bowl was hand rotated
    - D. Cold water used for mixing

46. A patient came for complete denture treatment. An alginate impression was made in the dry clinical atmosphere, left not poured and then poured after 24 hours. The resultant cast will be
    - A. Same dimension as that of the patient mouth
    - **B. Less in size than the patient' s mouth**
    - C. More in size than the patient's mouth
    - D. None of the above

47. A Complete Denture patient complained from loosening of the maxillary denture. How can you improve retention?
    A. The fit at the periphery region is adjusted to form a thick saliva film for retention
    B. The periphery region is adjusted to form thin saliva film for retention
    C. Porosity is provided in the posterior palatal region of the processed denture
    D. Porosity is provided in the anterior palatal region of the processed denture

48. A Mesio-Occlusal- Distal (MOD) amalgam restoration found fractured upon biting forces from the opposite natural tooth. What may the reason?
    A. Due to the brittleness of amalgam
    B. Due to ductility of amalgam
    C. Due to plasticity of amalgam
    D. Due to toughness of amalgam

49. A patient came to the clinic complaining about the denture cleaned in boiling water was no longer fitting in the patient mouth. Why?
    A. Patient did not keep the denture in the boiling water overnight
    B. Cleansing water temperature was higher than the glass transition temperature (Tg) of the resin
    C. Patient did not dry the denture after cleaning
    D. The cleansing water temperature was less than the glass transition temperature of the resin

50. Amalgam restoration was done opposing to a gold restoration in the patient mouth. After several months, the patient visited the clinic complaining that the amalgam restoration found discolored and corroded. Why?
    A. Dental amalgam is anodic to gold alloy

B. Dental amalgam cannot withstand oral environment for several months
C. Gold restoration cannot withstand pH of saliva for several months
D. Both dental amalgam and gold restoration were temporary restorative material

51. A 25 year old female patient wanted to improve the appearance of her anterior tooth. A ceramic veneering was prepared. The prepared veneer was found matching with shade guide but not with adjacent natural tooth. Why?
    A. Matching was not done under different lighting sources
    B. Shade guide matching was done under different lighting sources
    C. Ceramic veneering material lost its colour upon mixing
    D. Natural tooth lost its shade due to ceramic veneer adjacent to it

52. An additional silicone impression was poured by high strength stone in the dental laboratory. However, the cast could not reproduce all fine details of the cavity preparation. What might be the reason?
    A. Addition silicone used was hydrophilic
    B. Addition silicone is not compatible with high strength stone
    C. Additional silicone used was hydrophobic
    D. Addition silicone cannot be poured with gypsum materials

53. During the laboratory procedure, a dental technician found his Gold inlay casting made by lost wax technique rough. What may be the reason for it?
    A. Wax pattern was too large
    B. Wax pattern was too small
    C. Wax pattern surface was not smooth
    D. Wax pattern was painted with wetting agent

54. A patient came to the outpatient department for orthodontic treatment. Initially during the impression procedure, the alginate impression got distorted due to patient gagging. However later the dentist managed to make good impression. How?
    A. Excessive alginate is loaded only to the posterior portion of the tray and this region seated last
    B. A liquid consistency of the alginate is loaded on to the tray
    C. A regular setting alginate was selected
    D. Less alginate is loaded to the posterior portion and it was seated first

55. A gold alloy restoration was prepared. The restoration was found properly seating before cementation, but failed to seat when cemented with Glass Ionomer (GIC). One of the following reasons is not true for the current scenario
    A. Film thickness of the GIC was too high during cementation
    B. Too long time during completion of mixing and cementation
    C. Cement being placed on the tooth before being placed on the casting
    D. GIC cannot be used for cementation of gold alloy restoration

56. A post and core unit found detached in few days after cementation. What type of cement will be the best option for obtaining a root-cement-post and core unit that is bonded?
    A. Zinc oxide eugenol cement
    B. Dual cured resin cement
    C. Zinc poly carboxylate cement
    D. Calcium hydroxide cement

57. A patient approached the clinic with a fallen recent composite restoration. The pulp was protected with pulp protective zinc oxide eugenol cement. What may be the reason for failure of composite?
    A. Composite is a low strength material to restore
    B. Selected type of composite was not appropriate
    C. Zinc oxide eugenol was less strong
    D. Eugenol released from zinc oxide prevented the polymerization of composite resin

58. During an outreach clinical program for the school children, the dental graduate students suggested the use of fluoride varnishes than fluoride containing tooth pastes for children with early dental caries as "Fluoride varnishes can perform best compared to topical fluorides". One of the following is wrong with this statement
    A. Higher fluoride concentration in topical fluorides
    B. Higher fluoride concentration in fluoride varnishes
    C. Long exposure time for fluoride varnishes
    D. Less exposure time for topical varnishes

59. A posterior amalgam restoration was given for a patient with bruxism. Which factor may not contribute to wear and tarnish of the amalgam restoration after several years of placement?
    A. Slight condensation pressure applied while preparation
    B. Patient with high Sulphur containing diet
    C. A well- polished amalgam restoration surface
    D. Residual mercury content in the amalgam restoration

60. A class I amalgam restoration was finished chair side. What would be the best solution to store the scrap amalgam obtained after finishing procedure?
    A. Water
    B. Chloroform solution
    C. Agar gel solution
    D. Sodium thiosulfate solution

61. A PFM (Porcelain fused to metal) restoration was given for patient with large occlusal forces. However, the surface of the finished metal ceramic crown exhibited several dark inclusions. Which may not be the causative factor?
    - A. The metallic inclusions formed during grinding was not cleaned properly
    - **B. Core built up using metallic material**
    - C. Ceramics mixing spatula contaminated with metal shavings
    - D. Metallic instruments were employed for mixing ceramics

62. A 65 year old female patient was referred to endodontic department due to severe pain on her already restored teeth which lost part of its filling. One of the following is the biologically active material that may be used to promote periapical healing during the treatment
    - A. Corticosteroids
    - B. Zinc phosphate
    - **C. Mineral Trioxide Aggregate**
    - D. Zinc Polycarboxylate

63. A patient with 'Diastema' approached the dentist to improve his aesthetic appearance. What would be the ideal material for treating the current scenario?
    - A. PFM (Porcelain Fused to Metal restoration)
    - B. Aresin modified glass ionomer cement
    - **C. A composite restoration**
    - D. A zinc phosphate Cement

64. A completely edentulous patient without sufficient bone height and width was enthusiastic to have a dental implant instead of removable complete denture. What may be the treatment option?
    - A. Implant cannot be done and only complete denture is possible
    - **B. Grafting material may be tried to augment the bone deficiencies**
    - C. Stem cells can be transplanted to reduce the bone deficiency
    - D. Implant can be placed directly on the existing bone

65. An elastomeric impression was poured using dental stone. After some time, the poured model found slightly hot on touching. One of the following statements is true for this situation
    A. It is quite usual because heat is evolved during setting of dental stone
    B. It is because of the lower water to powder ratio
    C. Cast pouring should have been delayed
    D. Vacuum mixing may not be done

66. 60 years old patient attended your clinic with a complete denture of 15 years old complaining of inefficacy of mastication and ulceration at the angle of the mouth. The most common cause for of his complaining about mastication could be
    A. Decrease vertical dimension
    B. Increase vertical dimension
    C. The ulceration at the angle of his mouth
    D. Teeth wearing

67. A patient reported to the clinic after 3 months of implant surgery with firmly attached implant at the site of placement. This phenomena by which the bone adapts to the implant is known as
    A. Osteofixation
    B. Osseoadaptation
    C. Ossification
    D. Osseointegration

68. The patient, on whom an implant supported bridge is planned, is concerned about food lodgement beneath the prosthesis. What would you advise him regarding the most hygienic pontic design in an implant supported bridge?
    A. Sanitary pontic
    B. Ridge lap pontic
    C. Modified Ridge lap pontic
    D. Ovate pontic

69. The most advantageous aspect of implant supported FPD over a conventional FPD is that
    A. It is cheaper than conventional FPD
    B. It precludes no damage to the abutment teeth
    C. Requires no maintenance
    D. It provides superior strength with good hygiene

70. Using proper terminology is essential for communicating with the patient as well as the lab technician, what would you call the component of the implant assembly on which the prosthetic tooth is fixed?
    A. Retainer
    B. Denture
    C. Abutment
    D. Connector

71. Medical history of the patient requiring dental implant treatment in your clinic reveals that he is currently taking intravenous bisphosphonate therapy. You would
    A. Proceed as normal with the implant treatment
    B. Replace IV Bisphosphonate with Oral Bisphosphonate
    C. Check INR and proceed if normal
    D. Advice the patient against implant therapy at this stage

72. One of the most important factors in treatment planning for implant therapy is the quantity and quality of bone available. The most effective way to determine bone dimensions and density for treatment planning in implant treatment is
    A. Cone beam tomography
    B. Clinical bone mapping
    C. Radiograph
    D. Bimanual palpation of the ridge

73. A young adult patient consulted you about advantages of a resin retained FPD over an Implant to restore his missing lateral incisor. The following are the advantages of the resin retained bridge *except*
    A. Minimal or no preparation required
    B. Good aesthetics if ideal spacing exists
    C. Less expensive than conventional bridges and implants
    D. More durable than conventional bridge or implants

74. You want to clearly underline the advantages and indications of an implant supported prosthesis to your patient, who himself is quite inquisitive. All of the following can be considered as relative contraindications for implant therapy, *except*
    A. Severe parafunctional habits
    B. Uncontrolled diabetes
    C. High caries rate
    D. Smoking and poor oral hygiene

75. The young dentist shadowing the main dentist noticed that while recording the bite registration of the patient the dentist also made a protrusive bit record of the patient. What is the purpose of making a record of protrusive relation and what function does it serve after it is made?
    A. To register the condylar path and to adjust the inclination of the incisal guidance
    B. To aid in determining the freeway space and to adjust the inclination of the incisal guidance
    C. To register the condylar path and to adjust the condylar guides of the articulator so that they are equivalent to the condylar paths of the patient
    D. To aid in establishing the occlusal vertical dimension and to adjust the condylar guides of the articulator

76. During treatment planning for a case for full mouth rehabilitation the dentist decided that the occlusal vertical dimension of the patient would need to be increased. The main factor controlling a decision to increase the occlusal height of teeth for extensive oral reconstruction is whether
    A. The inter occlusal distance will be physiologically acceptable after treatment
    B. There will be sufficient tooth bulk in the abutment teeth for proper retention of the crowns
    C. At least two third of the original alveolar process will remain for adequate periodontal support
    D. The aesthetic appearance of the patient will improve sufficiently to warrant the planned reconstruction

77. Clinical and radiographic examination of the patient revealed less than ideal interproximal space required for placing implants. What are the criteria of space required for implant placement?
    A. Space should be at least as wide as the width of implant
    B. If the space required is less, more space can be created by interproximal stripping
    C. Implants placed next to natural teeth should allow an absolute minimum of 1 mm of intervening bone and preferably 2 mm
    D. If interproximal space is less than ideal, then a smaller diameter implant can be used in the first molar area with heavy functional loads

78. A sixteen year old boy reported to the clinic for replacing his upper right lateral incisor. What factor should be considered for treatment planning for implant placement in 'young' patients'?
    A. Minor patients cannot give consent for implant treatment, therefore implants are contraindicated
    B. Young patients do not have psychological maturity to accept implant therapy

C. Young patients may not be able to withstand surgical procedure of implant placement

D. Implant therapy should consider the effect of implants on jaw growth

79. After a thorough clinical examination of the completely edentulous patient, the dentist was of the opinion that an implant supported mandibular overdenture would be best suited for the patient. Which of the following are advantages of a mandibular implant overdenture as compared to a mandibular conventional denture?

A. Improved retention

B. Improved masticatory function

C. Improved quality of life

D. All of the above

80. Patient attitudes toward implant treatment are often vague due to lack of knowledge about the advantages of overdentures. Studies have shown that patient satisfaction after therapy is significantly higher in patients who receive mandibular overdentures versus conventional dentures. The main reason for the increased satisfaction is improved

A. Oral function

B. Aesthetics

C. Adaptation of the denture to the edentulous ridge

D. Proprioception

81. Maintaining good oral hygiene is important for the long-term success of implant therapy. Older patients typically have a more difficult time with maintenance of proper oral hygiene. It is recommended to check oral hygiene, plaque accumulation, and radiographic bone levels at each recall visit. Which of the following can result from the lack of proper plaque elimination from the implant-abutment surface?

A. Periimplantitis

B. Periodontitis

C. Pericoronitis
D. Gingivitis

82. A patient reported back to your clinic after few months with some 'problem' with his implant retained partial denture, the most common complication with Implant Retained Removable Partial Dentures is?
    A. Abutment tooth fracture
    B. Implant abutment loosening
    C. Framework warping
    D. Inflammation of the periimplant tissues

83. Studies have shown that implants can be placed even in young patients where the jaw growth has still not completed. Placement of dental implants in growing children has the lowest risk in which of the following region(s) of the mandible
    A. Molar regions
    B. Anterior region between mental foramina
    C. Premolar regions
    D. None of the above

84. A patient visited the clinic complaining of poor esthetics due to an uneven occlusal plane. Osseo integrated endosseous maxillary implants adjacent to the natural teeth might result in submerged implants due to the following *except*
    A. The continued eruption of the neighboring teeth
    B. The associated growth of the alveolus bone around implants
    C. The intrusion of implants
    D. None of the above

85. The mandibular left molars were determined to be non-restorable due to the extensive fracture. Implant restorations were selected to restore this area. When treatment planning for implant restoration, which of the following risk factor(s) is an absolute contraindication?

A. Diabetes
B. Osteoporosis
C. Hormone therapy
D. None of the above

86. A recent systematic review comparing the clinical outcomes of restored endodontically treated teeth with those of implant-supported restorations concluded that
    A. Survival rates of restored endodontically treated teeth and single implants did significantly differ
    B. The decision to treat a tooth endodontically or replace it with an implant must be based on factors other than the treatment outcomes of the procedures themselves
    C. Survival rates of restored endodontically treated teeth were higher
    D. Survival rates of single implants were higher

87. Concerning maxillary and mandibular posterior implants
    A. A 95% survival rate for mandibular implants and a 65–85% survival rate for maxillary implants are reported
    B. Bone quality and favorable loading are important factors for success of implant- supported restorations
    C. Minimum thickness of 1mm of surrounding bone is required for optimal osseointegration
    D. Stress to the implant is primarily affected by implant position

88. In considering all treatment options for a posterior edentulous area, a discussion of a removable partial denture ensues. Which of the following statements is correct regarding the choice between a removable partial dentures versus a fixed partial denture?
    A. Studies have shown that the survival rate of teeth adjacent to edentulous areas restored by removable partial dentures was greater than those replaced by nothing

B. Studies have shown that the survival rate of teeth adjacent to edentulous areas restored by fixed partial dentures was greater than those replaced by implant restorations
C. Studies have shown that the survival rate of teeth adjacent to edentulous areas restored by nothing was greater than those replaced by removable partial dentures
D. Studies have shown that the survival rate of teeth adjacent to edentulous areas restored by fixed partial dentures was greater than those replaced by removable partial dentures

89. The patient on whom an implant supported mandibular over denture is planned, is a heavy smoker. The effect of smoking on implant success and survival appeared to be more pronounced in
A. Type I bone
B. Type II bone
C. Type III bone
D. Type IV bone

90. The dentist and the lab technician were discussing the plan of occlusion for the complete denture patient. There commended occlusal concept for a conventional maxillary complete denture opposing mandibular implant-supported fixed complete denture is
A. Mutually protected occlusion
B. Canine guidance
C. Unilateral balanced occlusion
D. Bilateral balanced occlusion

91. A patient with para functional habits might report back to the clinic with certain complications. The most common signs of occlusal overload on implants are the following *except*
A. Screw loosening/fracture
B. Bone loss
C. Prosthesis fracture
D. Abutment fracture

92. A 50-year-old man due to recurrent adenoid cystic carcinoma underwent resection consisted of a left total maxillectomy. On the day of final insertion of the prosthesis. You will give all the following instructions regarding oral hygiene of obturator *except*
    A. When removed from the oral cavity, prostheses should be kept submerged in water to avoid distortion of the acrylic
    B. Removable prostheses should be removed while sleeping
    C. One should use a toothbrush to remove plaque from prostheses
    D. Prostheses should be worn 24 hours a day

93. On examination of a 35-year-old female, you find that the middle and posterior portions of the right maxilla were completely resected and there was a large defect involving the medial aspect of the right eye and nose. Maxillofacial prosthesis is, many a times, located in a highly visible facial area that is identified with one's identity. A successful rehabilitation of this patient with a maxillofacial prosthesis will benefit
    A. Esthetically
    B. Psychologically
    C. Functionally
    D. All of the above

94. You have rehabilitated a patient with definitive obturator for hemi-maxillectomy. You gave instructions on insertion, removal, and maintenance of the prosthesis. Which of the following items you will evaluate during the final insertion visit and the postinsertion follow - up visits
    A. Rest seats are fully seated and clasps are properly engaged
    B. Acrylic flanges are not overextended
    C. Occlusion is accurate
    D. All of the above items should be evaluated and monitored

95. A patient, living in northern region of Africa, received facial prosthesis to replace his nasal defect. He was exposed to factors like irradiation from sunlight, temperature, dust, perspiration. These factors will affect which quality of the prosthesis
    A. Retention
    B. Tissue healing
    C. Color stability
    D. Tissue preservation

96. A young male patient aged 18years presented to the Dental Teaching Hospital complaining of a swelling in the left maxillary posterior region. Clinical and radiographic examination was carried out. A biopsy was sent for investigation. The histopathologic result revealed an Odontogenic Myxoma involving the left maxillary posterior area. A surgeon planned to remove the tumor. In such situation the consultation from the Prosthodontist should be taken
    A. During the Surgery
    B. Before the surgery
    C. After the surgery
    D. No need of Prosthodontic consult

97. A 35-year-old female patient reported to the Department of Maxillofacial Rehabilitation with a defect in her right eye. The defect was caused by trauma due to a projectile injury during her childhood. On inspection, the sclera and iris were not completely present indicative of only the socket with the eye lids intact left behind. A maxillofacial prosthesis that artificially replaces an eye missing because of trauma, surgery or congenital absence and the prosthesis does not replace missing eyelids or adjacent skin, mucosa or muscle is called as
    A. Orbital Prosthesis
    B. Ocular Prosthesis
    C. Auricular Prosthesis
    D. Auxiliary Prosthesis

98. A 42 years old patient gave history of betel nut chewing habit for 20 years and restricted mouth opening in the last 10 years along burning mouth sensation to hot and spicy food. He underwent surgical procedure to treat restricted mouth opening problem. What is the name of this condition and, as a maxillofacial prosthodontist, which type of stent you will give to this patient?
    A. OSMF, Radiotherapy stent
    B. OSMF, Burn stent
    C. OSMF, Trismus stent
    D. OSMF, Paraplegic stent

99. A three years old child patient came to dental clinic accompanied with his parents and with chief complaint of speech difficulty due to cleft palate. What, in your opinion, is the main reason of speech difficulty in cleft palate patient?
    A. Difficulties in keeping the intraoral pressure
    B. Difficulties in keeping the extraoral pressure
    C. Difficulties in keeping the tongue pressure
    D. None of the above

100. The rehabilitation of a maxillofacial defect either congenital or acquired demands firm knowledge of the disease under treatment as well as mechanics and construction of the prosthetic device. Which of the following member of Maxillofacial rehabilitation team is a key member to attain it?
    A. Psychologist
    B. Surgeon
    C. Speech therapist
    D. Prosthodontist

101. As a team member of Maxillofacial rehabilitation team, you are planning to restore an intraoral defect with a definitive prosthesis. In your opinion, which type of occlusal scheme plays a very important

role and is favorable for comfort, function and longevity of the prosthesis?

A. Lingualized occlusion
B. Balanced occlusion
C. Non-balanced occlusion
D. Neutrocentic occlusion

102. As a member of maxillofacial rehabilitation team when you were asked to rehabilitate an auricular defect, which of the following procedure you will suggest to enhance the prosthetic prognosis while restoring auricular defect?

A. Retain the tragus
B. Avoid use of flaps with hair follicles
C. Defect must be lined with split thickness skin graft
D. All of the above

103. A 50 years old female visited dental Hospital with the complaint of pain after extraction of mandibular second premolar. She gave history of medication for osteoporosis, exposed & necrotic bone in the socket which has persisted for more than 8 weeks and no history of radiation therapy to the jaws. The condition was diagnosed as BRONJ. What does BRONJ stands for?

A. Bisphosphate- related osteonecrosis of the jaw
B. Bisphosphonate-related osteonecrosis of the jaw
C. Bioglass-related osteonecrosis of the jaw
D. Bicuspid- related osteonecrosis of the jaw

104. A patient visited to the dental clinic who had underwent hemi resection of the maxilla. On clinical examination you found that the defect is extended till the pharyngeal area. In such situation which type of obturator is fabricated?

A. Static
B. Functional
C. Meatus
D. None of the above

105. A 68-year-old male was referred from Department of Oncosurgery, Command Hospital, to department for prosthetic rehabilitation following partial rhinectomy of the right side of nose. Prosthodontic restoration of facial defect is a treatment of choice when surgical reconstruction is not possible. Which is the most common carcinoma that leads to partial or total rhinectomy?
    A. Squamous cell carcinoma
    B. Basal cell carcinoma
    C. Ameloblastoma
    D. Adenoid cystic carcinoma

106. A 50 years old edentulous patient had met with an accident and fractured his lower jaw in left posterior region. On radiographic examination it was found that the body of the mandible is fractured. The patient was not a denture wearer. Which type of Splint is fabricated for such patient to immobilize the jaw fracture?
    A. Gunning Splint
    B. Labiolingual Splint
    C. Kingsley Splint
    D. Fenestrated Splint

107. A patient underwent total maxillectomy due to carcinoma. In your opinion, which of the following provides best retention aids to fabricate large maxillofacial prosthesis that rest on movable tissue bed?
    A. Adhesives
    B. Magnets
    C. Undercuts
    D. Implants

108. For a 42 years old patient who has undergone hemi-maxillectomy 4 months before, you have planned to make a definitive obturator. While making final impression which of the landmark will be very useful in achieving best prognosis for the prosthesis

   A. Skin graft mucosa junction
   B. Soft tissue undercut
   C. Hard palate
   D. Remaining teeth

109. A young girl of 6 years age has congenital defect of cleft palate extending to soft palate. Her parents told that she has underwent three surgeries for closure of the extended cleft palate condition and now referred to the prosthodontist to fabricate a prosthesis. A prosthesis fabricated for this cleft palate patient is called as
   A. Appliance
   B. Obturator
   C. Speech aid prosthesis
   D. None of the above

110. Maxillofacial rehabilitation includes wide array of prosthesis, intraoral as well as extraoral prosthesis, that allows the patient to live as a functioning citizen within the society. In your opinion which of the following is not an intraoral prosthesis?
   A. Meatus obturator
   B. Ocular prosthesis
   C. Guiding plane prosthesis
   D. Gunning splint

111. Obturator is a prosthesis that is used to close the acquired defect. The word Obturator is derived from a Latin word 'obturare' which means
   A. To open up
   B. To shut off
   C. To shift up
   D. To swift off

112. The oral cancer patient has undergone irradiation treatment modality. The patient was informed about the side effects. Which of the following is the most significant side effect when patients with oral

and pharyngeal tumors are irradiated for cure and which might in turn affect the prognosis of the final maxillofacial prosthesis?

A. Osteointegration
B. Osteoporosis
C. Osteoradionecrosis
D. Osteonecrosis

113. A patient undergone right side condyle resection is able to achieve an appropriate mediolateral position of the mandible but is unable to repeat this position consistently for mastication. Which of the following prosthesis you will fabricate for this patient?

A. Gunning splint
B. Stent
C. Guide flange
D. Obturator

114. One of your Oral surgeon friend who is a member of maxillofacial rehabilitation discuss with you about number of hemi maxillectomy and mandibulectomy cases he does in their hospital. He told you that the most common cause for an unfortunate situation of acquired maxillary or mandibular defect is

A. Dental cyst
B. Accidents
C. Carcinoma
D. All of the above

115. You have made an impression of an auricular defect for a patient and sent it to your routine dental laboratory. The dental technician is not trained in maxillofacial prosthesis fabrication and asks for your help. Which methods you will teach the technician for fabrication of ear wax/clay pattern: i. Donor method ii. Mirror image method iii. Inversion method. iv. Boxing method?

A. i, iii, iv
B. iii, iv

C. i, ii
D. ii, iii, iv

116. The parents of 3 days old baby with cleft lip and palate came to the dental clinic, saying that they were referred by the pediatrician. It was decided to give feeding plate to the child. In the current protocol followed for the treatment for cleft lip and cleft palate, Naso-alveolar molding is done from
    A. Birth to 6 weeks
    B. Birth to 8 weeks
    C. Birth to 10 weeks
    D. Birth to 12 weeks

117. A patient by name Moalla came to a prosthodontist for prosthesis, on intraoral examination it was found that lower molar crown was root canal treated and needs crown and patient insisted on gold crown. Which of the following marginal designs is theoretically the best finishing margin for cast gold restorations, allowing and adaptation of the gold to the tooth?
    A. Shoulder
    B. Shoulder with a bevel
    C. Chamfer
    D. Bevel or feather edge

118. Mostafa, a complete denture patient after delivery of the prostheses returns after 3 weeks complaining of speech problems especially with the "s" sounds, which sounds like "th". What could be the cause?
    A. Teeth are placed too buccally
    B. Insufficient vertical dimension of occlusion
    C. Incisor teeth set too far palatally
    D. This is part of normal adaptation process

119. A female patient during the delivery of the denture appointment, complains that the “bite doesn’t feel right”. What should be done to this?
    A. Use an articulating paper and adjust intraorally
    B. Remove the denture and apply topical anesthetic
    C. Ask him to bite forcefully until he achieves occlusion
    D. Perform a lab or a clinical remount for further occlusal equilibration

120. Patient by name Sultan came with a chief complaint of missing teeth. On intraoral examination it was found maxillary complete edentulousness and mandibular Kennedy’s class I situation. What occlusal scheme should be given in this patient?
    A. Canine guided
    B. Bilateral balanced
    C. Unilateral balanced
    D. Cross articulation

121. Patient by name Farooq comes with missing upper anterior teeth. The teeth arrangement in this case should be arranged based on esthetics and phonetics. Their position typically should be
    A. Lingual to the ridge
    B. Exactly over the ridge
    C. Facial to the ridge
    D. 3mm above the ridge

122. A complete edentulous patient comes to the OPD for replacement of his teeth. How residual ridge resorption can be minimized when fabricating a complete denture?
    A. Soaking dentures in hot water prior to use
    B. Always using bilateral balanced occlusal scheme
    C. Appropriate adjustment of denture occlusion post-insertion
    D. Use of denture adhesive to ensure proper retention of denture

123. A partial edentulous patient comes for replacement of teeth. Common complication with implant retained removable partial denture is
    A. Framework warpage
    B. Inflammation of peri-implant tissue
    C. Abutment tooth fracture
    D. Implant abutment loosening

124. A patient by name Abdulla came to college of Dentistry clinic for replacement of his missing teeth. On thorough intraoral examination, treatment plan include a distal extension partial denture. Which of the following is considered the least favorable choice of retainer in a distal extension removable partial denture design?
    A. I bar
    B. Embrassure clasp
    C. Aker's clasp
    D. Wrought wire clasp

125. A patient came for replacement of missing teeth. What is the minimal acceptable crown/prosthesis-to- root ratio for planning a fixed partial denture?
    A. 1:2
    B. 1:3
    C. 1:1
    D. 1:4

126. A patient by name Hussain wants to get treatment done for his discolored upper anterior teeth. He wants minimal invasive procedure. Which of the following occlusal relationships may pose a contraindication for placement of a porcelain laminate veneer (PLV) restoration?
    A. Anterior open bite
    B. Class I occlusion

C. Class II occlusion

D. Edge-to-edge anterior tooth relationship

127. Patient has come for replacement of missing teeth. Treatment option was to give a fixed partial denture. Tooth preparation was done and impression made. During metal try-in stage the dentist wants to choose the shade for the patient. The ideal condition during shade selection

A. Using a corrective light source that burns at 5,500^0 K

B. Choosing final shades on sunny days only

C. Using a corrective light source that burns at 4,500^0 K

D. Using only composite shade guide

128. Patient came to Jouf dental clinic with severe pain on his lower posterior tooth. After emergency patient care, which of the following treatment sequences is recommended?

A. Preparation and provisionalization only

B. Crown-lengthening procedure, endodontics, and then preparation and provisionalization

C. Crown-lengthening procedure, preparation and provisionalization

D. Mount study casts, diagnostic wax-up, preparation and provisionalization

129. A patient by name Anwar came to department of prosthodontics for treatment of his fractured central incisor. On clinical and radiographic examination there was no sufficient remaining tooth structure to adequately retain a restoration. What is the best treatment option in this case?

A. Cut in retention channels

B. Use pins to aid in the buildup of the core

C. **Prophylactic endodontic treatment should be considered**

D. No additional treatment is needed

130. In restoring a patient with all-ceramic restoration, which of the following statements is accurate regarding cementation technique?
    A. Cement shades change color after cementation
    B. Cement shades do not affect the shade of the final restoration
    C. **The luting cement can cause a perceptible color difference in the final restoration**
    D. Cement shades change color in the presence of moisture

131. Patient of age 24 by name Mohammed has come to college of Dentistry to enhance his smile. On clinical examination, it was found that there is a decrease in clinical crown length. One of the treatment options is orthodontic extrusion to increase the crown height. A possible benefit with orthodontic eruption of anterior teeth is
    A. Creating a more favorable crown-to-root ratio
    B. Exposing a less stained root surface area that is more esthetic
    C. **Minimal scar tissue formation**
    D. Creating tighter root proximity

132. An edentulous patient has slight undercuts on both tuberosities and also on the facial of the anterior maxilla. To construct a satisfactory maxillary complete denture, you should reduce which of the following?
    A. **All undercuts**
    B. The anterior undercut only
    C. Both tuberosity undercuts
    D. None of them

133. If a patient comes to dental clinic, which of the following is the most important reason for treatment of hyperplastic tissue before construction of a complete or removable partial denture?
    A. To feel the patient better
    B. To make the face-bow transfer easier
    C. To make the final impression material flow better
    D. **To provide firm, stable base for the denture**

134. Patient by name Salah 50 years old came to department of Prosthodontics for treatment. On intraoral examination, there are multiple carious teeth, missing teeth, supra-eruption and drifting of few teeth. Dentist wants to make a Face-bow record. So, the condylar guidance is a factor which
   A. **Is totally dictated by the patient**
   B. Is totally controlled by the dentist
   C. Is partially dictated by the patient and partially adjusted by the dentist
   D. Can be adjusted by the laboratory technician

135. A female patient has visited a dental clinic. On clinical examination, it was found that right canine needs a conservative tooth preparation. The prosthodontist planned to give a $3/4^{th}$ crown. What should be the path of insertion for an anterior 3/4 crown?
   A. **Be parallel to the incisal 1/2 to 2/3 of the labial surface rather than the long axis of the tooth**
   B. Be perpendicular to the incisal 1/2 of the labial surface rather than the long axis of the tooth
   C. Be parallel to the long axis of the tooth
   D. Be parallel to the cervical 1/3 of the labial surface rather than the long axis of the tooth

136. A patient of high esthetic demand needs a fixed partial denture. What pontic design would you use in such patient when preparing upper anterior teeth for fixed partial denture?
   A. Ovate pontic
   B. Saddle ridge lap pontic
   C. **Modified ridge lap pontic**
   D. Sanitary pontic

137. Patient by name Mohammed has visited a dental clinic for replacement of his missing upper teeth. On examination, he needs upper complete denture. In this patient what should be kept in mind in recording the posterior palatal seal in upper denture?
   A. Is placed 3mm posterior to the vibrating line
   B. Is not necessary when fabricating a complete denture on a patient with a flat palate
   C. **Will vary in outline and depth according to the palatal form of the patient**
   D. Is not necessary if a metal base is used

138. A complete denture patient has come for removable prosthesis. Upper complete denture was planned for that patient. Which of the following landmarks is least relevant to the location of the posterior palatal seal area?
   A. Vibrating line
   B. Fovea palatinae
   C. **Hamular process**
   D. Pterygomaxillary notch

139. A complete edentulous patient has come to a dental centre. Complete denture was planned and denture fabrication was done and delivered to patient. At the first appointment after insertion of complete dentures, the presence of generalized soreness on the crest of the mandibular ridge is most likely due to
   A. Defective tissue registration
   B. **Premature occlusal contacts**
   C. The newness of the denture
   D. Incomplete polymerization of the denture base

140. A patient by name Sultan came to college of Dentistry, Jouf University. He needs full mouth rehabilitation. A plaster index is made and used to
    A. Maintain bite registration
    B. Maintain the vertical dimension of occlusion
    C. **Preserve the face-bow transfer**
    D. No need of plaster index

141. A female patient of high esthetic expectation has visited Dental clinic. On intraoral examination, she needs a smile makeover. In establishing esthetic outcomes for the anterior maxilla, "golden proportion" is followed which relates to the width of the teeth. The ratio is
    A. **1:1.618**
    B. 1:3.14
    C. 1:1
    D. 1:2

REFERENCES

Anusavice K. J., Chiayi Shen and Palph Rawls. 2012. *Phillips' Science of Dental materials*. 12th ed. Saunders.

Anusavice, Kenneth J. 1996. *Phillip's Science of Dental Materials.* 9th ed. Philadelphia: W.B. Saunders.

Babbush, Charles A., Jack A. Hahn, Jack T. Krauser, and Joel L. Rosenlicht. 2011. *Dental Implants: The Art and Science.* 2nd Edition. Saunders publisher.

Carr, Alan B., Brown. David T. 2015. *McCracken's Removable Partial Prosthodontics* 13th Ed. Mosby Publisher.

Combe E. C. 1992. *Notes on Dental Materials.* 6th ed. Edinburgh: New York. Churchill Livingstone.

Gladwin, M., Bagby, M. 2004. *Clinical Aspects of Dental Materials.* 2nd ed.

Malone, W. F. P. 1997. *Tylman's Theory and Practice of Fixed Prosthodontics,* 8th ed. AIPD Publishers.

McCabe, J. F. 2008. *Applied Dental Materials.* 9th ed. Wiley-Blackwell.

Misch, Carl E. 2008. *Contemporary Implant Dentistry.* 3rd Ed. Mosby: Elsevier.

Rahn, Arthur O., Charles M., Jr. Heartwell. 2011. *Textbook of Complete Dentures.* 5th Ed. Pmph USA Ltd.

Rosenstiel, Stephen, Land, Martin and Fujimoto. 2015. *Contemporary Fixed Prosthodontics.* 5th Ed. Elsevier publishing Co.

Sakaguchi, Ronald, Ferracane, Jack andPowers, John. 2018. *Restorative Dental Materials* 14th ed. Elsevier.

Shillingburg Herbert T. et al., 2012. *Fundamentals of Fixed Prosthodontics,* 4th Ed. Quintessence Publisher.

Winkler, Sheldon. 2015. *Essentials of Complete Denture Prosthodontics,* 2nd Ed.India: AITBS Publishers.

Zarb, George A. 2012. *Prosthodontic Treatment for Edentulous Patients: Complete Dentures and Implant-Supported Prostheses.* 13th Ed. Mosbypublisher.

In: Scenario Based MCQ in Dentistry ISBN: 978-1-53617-298-0
Editors: M. Khursheed Alam et al. © 2020 Nova Science Publishers, Inc.

Chapter 9

SCENARIO BASED MCQS IN PEDODONTICS

Ravi Kumar Gudipaneni, MDS,
Josna Vinutha Yadiki, MDS and Darrel Singh, MDS
Pedodontics, Preventive Dentistry Department, College of Dentistry,
Jouf University, Aljouf, Saudi Arabia

This chapter has been primarily written for the benefit of under graduate dental students, students appearing for postgraduate exams and various professional licensing examinations to broaden their knowledge and understanding of clinical pediatric dentistry.

A problem-solving approach has been adopted since the dental students need to analyze and interpret various clinical scenarios and it allows students to develop their skills in the management and effective solutions. Problem solving is a core skill, which the dental undergraduate must develop and refine for examinations and help the students to apply their knowledge into a clinically useful format. This chapter tries to cover a variety of problem-solving questions in the field of pediatric dentistry most of which are examiner favorites. We have attempted to cover a wide variety of MCQs and clinical scenario questions, featuring around 150 problem-based questions that demonstrate many of the problems commonly seen in the field of pediatric dentistry and offers practice for the students to solve problem-based questions. More emphasis has been given to areas such as pediatric endodontics and children with special health care needs. There is a combination of questions with some required straight forward recognition and others requiring the application of knowledge. Hopefully, this will be a good revision and aid to those undergoing examination.

Therefore, this chapter is designed to address a range of common clinical problems encountered in paediatric dental practice. Intended primarily for the undergraduate, we hope this chapter provides good practice to solve various problem based MCQS and will also be of value to the junior postgraduate and to those preparing for competitive examinations.

1. When primary molars are prepared for stainless steel crowns should the depth for reduction of the proximal surface be similar to the depth of the buccal and lingual surfaces?
    A. Yes; reduction of all wall is similar for best retention
    B. **No, proximal reduction is greater to allow the crown to pass the contact area**
    C. No, the buccal surfaces have the greatest reduction to remove the cervical bulge
    D. Yes, all undercuts are uniformly removed so that the steel crown can be seated

2. Eight (8) year old child who has sustained a fracture of maxillary permanent central incisor in which 2mm of the pulp is exposed; presents for treatment three hours after injury. Which of the following should be considered?
    A. **Remove the surface 1-2 mm of pulp tissue and place calcium hydroxide**
    B. Place calcium hydroxide directly on the exposed pulp
    C. Pulpotomy using formocresol
    D. Pulpectomy and immediate root filling

3. A healthy 6-year-old child presents with carious maxillary second primary molar with a necrotic pulp. Which treatment would be preferred?
   A. Extraction
   B. Indirect pulp treatment
   C. Pulpotomy
   D. **Pulpectomy**

4. 8-year-old child presents with all permanent incisors erupted, but yet only three permanent first molars are erupted. Oral examination reveals a large gingival bulge in the unerupted permanent area. A panoramic radiograph shows the alveolar emergence of the un-erupted permanent first molar crown and three fourth tooth developments, there are no other radiographic abnormalities. The most appropriate diagnosis and treatment plan in such situation would be?
   A. Dentigerous cyst; surgical enucleation.
   B. Ankylosis of the molar, removal of the first molar to allow the second one to erupt into its place.
   C. Ankylosis of the molar, surgical soft tissues exposure and luxation of the molar
   D. Idiopathic failure of eruption, surgical soft tissues exposure

5. 12-year-old child presents with symptoms of widespread gingivitis with bleeding and general malaise for several weeks. How would you manage this patient?
   A. Prescribe Metronidazole 100mg
   B. Locally debride, give oral hygiene instruction and prescribe H_2O_2 mouth wash.
   C. Give a prophylaxis with ultra-sonic scaling
   D. **Refer for hematological screening**

6. A 12-year-old girl complains of sore mouth, she has painful cervical lymphadenitis and a temperature of 39°c, oral examination shows numerous yellow grey lesions. What is the MOST LIKELY diagnosis?
   A. Measles
   B. Erythema multiform
   C. **Herpetic gingivostomatitis**
   D. Stevens-Johnson syndrome

7. An upper deciduous molar has a caries exposure and on X ray the corresponding 2nd permanent premolar is absent. What treatment would you do to the deciduous tooth?
   A. Pulpotomy
   B. **Endodontic treatment**
   C. Pulp capping
   D. Extraction

8. A seven-year-old boy fell of his bicycle 2 weeks ago and broke his maxillary central incisor. The pulp horn is visible as a pin point. The tooth is vital. What would be your treatment will be?
   A. Pulpectomy
   B. Place calcium hydroxide and fill with composite resin
   C. **Calcium hydroxide pulpotomy**
   D. Apexification/RCT

9. A 10-year-old boy presents with small greyish white lesion surrounded by a red halo on the soft palate and tonsillar pillars, small vesicles are found. He has fever and pain in the ear. The MOST probable diagnosis is
   A. **Herpangina**
   B. Herpetic gingiva stomatitis
   C. Mumps
   D. Aphthous ulcers

10. A patient has improperly formed DEJ (Dentino Enamel Junction), reduction in size of pulp chamber, chipping and attrition of enamel that would be the condition mostly
    A. Fluorosis
    B. Amelogenesis imperfecta
    C. **Dentinogenesis imperfecta**
    D. Hyoplasia

11. Which of the following should be made in the proximal occlusal cavity preparation for amalgam in deciduous teeth compared to permanent ones
    A. The occlusal lingual walls need not to be extended to self-cleansing areas
    B. **It is necessary to include fissures in the occlusal outline**
    C. The lingual angle should be sharper
    D. The axio-pulpal line angle should not be bevelled

12. Which of the following anomalies occurs during the initiation and proliferation stages of tooth development?
    A. Amelogenesisimperfecta
    B. Dentinogenesisimperfecta
    C. Enamel hypoplasia
    D. **Oligodontia**

13. A child has sustained a traumatic exposure of primary central incisor, he presents to you for treatment two days after the injury. Which of the following should be considered?
    A. Pulpotomy and Ca(OH)2
    B. Pulpotomy and formocresol
    C. Direct pulp capping
    D. **Pulpectomy**

14. A 5-year-old boy had extraction of 75 due to badly decay. The MOST common consequence arising from premature extraction of deciduous molars is
    A. **Loss of arch length**
    B. Loss of speech sound
    C. Loss of facial contour
    D. Loss of vertical height

15. A 4-year-old boy has been referred to pediatric dentist. The most common reason to refer a child to a Pedodontist is problem with
    A. Rampant caries
    B. **Behaviour management**
    C. Endodontic treatments in primary teeth
    D. Space maintainers

16. A patient suffers a blow to his maxillary central incisor without resulting in fracture. The status of would be pulp…?
    A. Immediate necrosis
    B. Becomes non-vital but only if treatment is delayed too long
    C. **Becomes non vital irrespective of treatment**
    D. No changes are seen later if fracture does not occur

17. At birth, the oral cavity of new born baby usually contains
    A. S. mutans only
    B. **No microorganism**
    C. S. mutans and S. salivarius
    D. Lactobacilli and S. mutans

18. A patient 8- years old has 3 of first premolars erupted with swelling on the ridge of the unerupted premolar. X ray shows a fully developed crown and ¾ roots development with no other pathology. What is your management?
    A. Remove the dentigerous cyst
    B. **Soft tissues incision to allow eruption**

C. Soft tissues incison accompanied with orthodontic appliance to help with eruption
D. Extraction

19. Child with less than normal number of teeth, mandibular lateral incisor is larger than usual; on x rays it shows with two roots and two roots canals; your diagnosis is?
    A. Gemination
    B. **Fusion**
    C. Concrescence
    D. Taurodontism

20. A 10- year old child presents with crowding of the dentition and desires correction. What your first step would be…?
    A. **Perform mixed dentition analysis**
    B. Extract the deciduous teeth
    C. Ask the patient to come after the deciduous teeth fall off and complete permanent dentition erupts
    D. Apply a fixed appliance

21. An 8-year old child, on examination you find 75 with carious exposure. On X-ray you find 35 missing. Your treatment is:
    A. Extraction of 75 allowing 36 to move mesially
    B. **Pulpotomy on 75 and wait indefinitely**
    C. Extraction of 75 and place a fixed space retainer to be replaced with fixed bridge.
    D. Extraction of 65 and 75

22. Several application has been suggested to increase the effectiveness of prophylactic application of topical fluoride which include all *except* -
    A. Increase Fluoride ions in solution “increase concentration”
    B. **Increase PH of fluoride**
    C. Increase exposure time to topical fluoride
    D. Pre-treat enamel with 0.5% phosphoric acid

23. Which is the right sequence of the histological stages of tooth development
    A. **Initiation, proliferation, histodifferentiation, morphodifferentiation, mineralization**
    B. Proliferation, initiation, histodifferentiation, morphodifferentiation, mineralization
    C. Proliferation, morphodifferentiation, histodifferentiation, mineralization
    D. Initiation, proliferation, morphodifferentiation, histodifferentiation, mineralization

24. A 10-year-old boy presents with a non-vital, non-mobile tooth. What would be the treatment is?
    A. Pulpectomy with calcium hydroxide
    B. Pulpectomy with Zinc oxide eugenol
    C. Pulpotomy with formocresol
    D. **No treatment is required if tooth is asymptomatic**

25. At birth, some calcified dental tissues are presented
    A. All deciduous teeth and all permanent incisors
    B. All deciduous teeth and permanent central incisors
    C. **All deciduous teeth and the first permanent molars**
    D. Deciduous teeth

26. A 5-year-old child who has been diagnosed with hyperkinesis appears at your office in an obvious state of anxiety at the impeding treatment. Upon interview, his mother relates that he is taking 30 mg of methylphenidate (Ritalin) daily. Which of the following should you do in planning to make the child more manageable?
    A. Double the dose of Ritalin 1 hour before the dental appointment
    B. ask the mother to discontinue medication on the day of dental visit
    C. balance the medication with 65mg of Phenobarbital

D. **call the child's physician and discuss with him the child's drug regimen**

27. An 8 - year-old boy is referred by a pediatric neurologist for dental treatment. His mother narrates the following history: At present he is receiving daily dose of an amphetamine. His teacher complains the he never pays attention. He is left handed and a bit clumsy. The most probable behavior disorders this patient demonstrates is -
    A. Autism
    B. Epilepsy
    C. **Hyperkinesis**
    D. Mental retardation

28. A mother and her 4-year-old son are seated alone in a reception area with the child staring off into space and continuously twisting a strand of hair about his fingers. Upon entry of another person, the child began to beat his fist against the side of his face and behaves as though he does not hear his mother speaking to him. This behavior is most characteristic of
    A. **Child with autism**
    B. An overprotected child
    C. A mentally retarded child
    D. First dental appointment anxiety

29. A 7 - year- old patient has an end on molar relation and normal vertical and horizontal overlap. The mandibular lateral incisors are erupting slightly lingually. What would be the treatment choice?
    A. **Lingual arch space maintainer**
    B. Refer to orthodontist
    C. Continue routine dental care and developmental supervision
    D. Myofunctional therapy

30. In a child with a suspected diagnosis of leukemia and with a badly infected primary teeth, the procedure of choice would be -
    A. administer antibiotics and refer the patient to physician
    B. **obtain consultation before determining the course of action**
    C. obtain a blood account, admit the child to a hospital for extraction
    D. provide palliative only

31. A 12-year-old child is 30 inches tall and has excellent body proportions. Laboratory studies are likely to reveal which of the following conditions.
    A. Hypothyroidism
    B. **Hypopituitarism**
    C. Malabsorption syndrome
    D. Adrenogenital syndrome

32. A 9-year-old epileptic patient has a petitmal seizure in the office. No other member of the office staff is available to render assistance. The proper course of management is to
    A. administer oxygen
    B. inject barbiturate
    C. **wait until the episode passes**
    D. call the local emergency code for assistance

33. A 12-year-old boy who is an athlete, broke his upper right incisor during a practice session 2 days back. Almost half of the clinical crown is fractured. Which of the following is the least preferred treatment for this patient.
    A. Pulpectomy and obturation, wait and watch
    B. **Pulpectomy, obturation and post and core to restore the crown**
    C. Pulpectomy, obturation followed by stainless steel crown with window.
    D. Extraction

34. A dentist notices a rash on a child's wrist while treating carious tooth. Upon enquiry the child says the he was wearing a metal bracelet in that region. Which type of crown should he use for restoring this tooth?
    A. **procera all ceramic crown**
    B. porcelain fused to metal
    C. stainless steel crown
    D. resin bonded FPD

35. An adolescent had malaligned teeth in the maxillary anterior region due to a congenitally missing left central incisor. Treatment with a fixed prosthesis was planned after orthodontic repositioning and de-rotation of the teeth. Which restoration is least preferred?
    A. Metal ceramic crown
    B. All ceramic crown
    C. **Cantilever pontic**
    D. Resin bonded prosthesis

36. A removable appliance with a clasp on the primary maxillary canine was used to replace missing posterior teeth in a child when he was 4 years old. Approximately at what age of the child should this clasp be removed from the primary canine?
    A. 5 years
    B. **7 years**
    C. 9 years
    D. 11 years

37. A patient aged 12 years reports with a swelling in the left mandibular premolar region. Radiographically there is a well circumscribed, unilocular radiolucent lesion where the first premolar failed to develop and there was no history of extraction before. The probable diagnosis is
    A. Dentigerous cyst
    B. Primordial cyst
    C. Odontogenickeratocyst
    D. **Eruption cyst**

38. The classical triad of multiple punched out radiolucent lesions of membranous bone, exopthalmous and diabetes insipidus is characteristic of
    A. Hand- Schuller-Christian diseases
    B. Eosinophilic granuloma
    C. **Letterer- Siwe disease**
    D. Histioctosis Y

39. In a 10- year old girl, a large radiolucent area was detected radiographically in the apical region of permanent mandibular incisors. They tested vital. The lesion was asymptomatic. When the lesion was explored surgically it revealed a large, nonlined, hollow space containing a few cobweb- like fibers and a small pool of dark reddish fluid. Most probably the diagnosis is
    A. central fibroma
    B. A ranula
    C. **A traumatic or hemorrhagic bone cyst**
    D. A chronic periapical lesion

40. Ina 7-year -old child small, irregular, bright red spots on the buccal mucosa, with bluish-white specks in the centers, may be seen at the onset of
    A. Mumps
    B. Herpes
    C. Rubella
    D. **Rubeola**

41. In a child, a combination of malnutrition, steatorrhea, chronic respiratory function, thyroid deficiency, a great slat loss through skin and functional disturbances in secretory mechanism of various glands is indicative of
    A. **cystic fibrosis**
    B. pierre robin syndrome
    C. herediatry fructose intolerance
    D. immune deficiency syndrome

42. An 8 - year- old girl is admitted to the hospital for treatment of "swollen gums" of three weeks' duration. Oral examination reveals markedly edematous and erythematous gingivae. Her parents state that the child has been well although, in the past month, some malaise, anorexia and occasional fever were noted. The most appropriate course of action is to
    A. Refer a child to a periodontist
    B. **Request a hematologic consultation**
    C. Prescribe a 10 -day course of oral penicillin/metronidazole
    D. Enroll the child in an active prevention programme that emphasis adequate home care.

43. Bitewing radiographs of a 5 - year- old child show interproximal caries just short of the dentinoenamel junction. The dentist should recommend.
    A. **Restoration of the teeth as soon as possible**
    B. prophylaxis and topical fluoride application
    C. disking of affected area
    D. three-month recall for re- evaluation

44. If a successful pulpotomy cannot be accomplished in a 5 -year -old child with a chronically infected primary molar, which of the following is the most acceptable treatment.
    A. treat with an antibiotic and allow the tooth to remain in place
    B. allow the tooth to remain in the mouth as a space maintainer
    C. allow the tooth to remain in the mouth unless it is creating pain for the patient
    D. **extract the tooth to prevent damage to the surrounding bone and developing permanent tooth**

45. Following removal of a relatively large area of decay in recently erupted permanent molar, an exposure of the pulpal tissue is noted. The dentist decided to perform a puloptomy using calcium hydroxide to treat the tissue remaining in the root canals. The dentist would expect a dentin bridge to form at
    A. **A level somewhat below the amputation**
    B. A level halfway between the apex and the amputation
    C. The exact level of amputation
    D. The apical site

46. A healthy 5-year old child has a necrotic pulp in a primary second molar that has a permanent successor. The primary second molar should be
    A. **treated endodontically**
    B. allowed to remain in the mouth, unless it is creating pain for the patient
    C. allowed to remain in the mouth, but treated with an antibiotic to eliminate infection
    D. drained through an opening through the crown into the pulp chamber, but allowed to remain in the mouth to serve as a space maintainer.

47. A healthy 8-year-old child has a fractured permanent central incisor. The pulp is widely exposed and vital. From radiographs, root ends appear incompletely calcified. The recommended procedure is to
    A. cap the pulp
    B. extract the tooth
    C. **perform puloptomy**
    D. remove the entire pulp.

48. A 9 -year-old child reports to the office with a maxillary permanent central incisor having a small hypoplastic spot on the labial surface as the chief complaint. The child gives a history of fall when he was 4

year old, which resulted in a fracture of his maxillary primary incisor. The most probable diagnosis.

A. hypoplasia due to systemic disease
B. Fluorosis
C. **Turners tooth**
D. amelogenesis imperfecta

49. When a permanent tooth is intruded, the tendency for the injury to be followed by rapid root resorption, pulp necrosis or ankylosis is greater. To prevent this, pulp tissue is extirpated and calcium hydroxide is placed inside the root canal as an interim dressing. This is usually done

A. **Within 2 weeks after the injury**
B. within 6 weeks after the injury
C. immediately after the trauma
D. within 8 weeks after the injury

50. A 9-year -old boy has a traumatized permanent central incisor with a pulp exposure of 2 mm in diameter. The injury occurred 4 weeks ago; the tooth now has a necrotic pulp. Radiographs shows that the root has developed to two-thirds of its length and has a wide open apex. No other significant signs and symptoms exist. Treatment of choice is to

A. Extract the tooth and place a prosthesis
B. **induce apexification and fill the root canal**
C. fill the root canal and place a retrograde amalgam
D. Orthodontic traction

51. A child of 7 years comes to the dental clinic for routine checkup. Upon history taking it is revealed that one year back the child's family had shifted to a place where the fluoride content in the water is 3ppm. Which of his teeth will be affected by fluorosis

A. None of the teeth
B. First Molars
C. **Third molars**
D. Incisors and canines

52. The child who misbehaves in the dental office during the first appointment: 1 is often the innocent victim of circumstances, 2 will bear a grudge if the dentist forces him or her to behave, 3 looks upon the dentist as a symbol and displeasure towards the dentist is not personal
    A. 1 and 2
    B. 2 and 3
    C. **1 and 3**
    D. 1, 2 and 3

53. During dental examinations on ten-year-old children which permanent tooth surface would show the highest carious or filled prevalence?
    A. Mesial surface of the central incisors
    B. Occlusal surface of the first premolar
    C. Labial surface of the canine
    D. **Occlusal surface of the first molar**

54. There are hard dark brown lesions on the labial surfaces of all four primary cuspids in a seven-year-old child. The teeth are not painful and scraping with a spoon excavator yields only a few flecks of dry discolored dentin. What are these lesions
    A. Active carious lesions
    B. **Arrested carious lesions**
    C. Local enamel hypoplasia
    D. Abrasion

55. A 6 year old child is examined for carious leions. What is the order in which caries usually develops in the Occlusal and proximal surfaces of second primary molars
    A. First – mesial; second – Occlusal; third – distal
    B. First – occlusal; second – distal; third – mesial
    C. **First – Occlusal; second – mesial; third – distal**
    D. First – mesial; second – distal; third – mesial

56. A child of 5 years of age reports for a routine checkup. What is the earliest appearance of carious demineralization of the enamel that can be detected clinically?
    A. **An opaque white area that is hard to the explorer tip**
    B. A chalky white area that can be penetrated by pressure from an explorer tip
    C. A dark brown area that resists penetration by an explorer
    D. Cavitation of the enamel surface that appears radiolucent on the radiograph

57. A child 12 years old reports with a maxillary anterior diastema. With the eruption of which teeth do maxillary anterior diastema normally close
    A. First molars
    B. Third molars
    C. Premolars
    D. **Canines**

58. A 4-year-old child reported to the dental clinic with less than a normal number of erupted teeth and presence of bifid shaped lateral incisor. Upon radiographic evaluation the bifid lateral incisor showed the presence of two roots and two root canals. What is the probable diagnosis?
    Dilacerations
    A. Concrescence
    B. **Fusion**
    C. Gemination

59. While performing restorative procedures on a deciduous tooth in a 4 year old child it is important to know that the thickness of the dentin in primary teeth as compared to the permanent teeth is
    A. 1/4
    B. 1/3
    C. 1/2
    D. **2/3**

60. A child aged 3 reports to the dental clinic for dental checkup. Upon history taking the mother reveals that the child has the habit of night time bottle feeding. Which primary teeth are most likely to get severely decayed?
    - A. Maxillary molars
    - B. Maxillary and mandibular canines
    - C. Mandibular incisors
    - D. **Maxillary incisors**

61. While examining a preschool child it is found out that the child is suffering from generalized acute gingival inflammation. The most common cause
    - A. Vitamin C deficiency
    - B. **Acute herpetic gingivostomatitis**
    - C. Drug therapy
    - D. Acute necrotizing gingivitis

62. Upon examination of a 2-year-old child an eruption cyst is found in the region of second molar. What is the treatment of choice?
    - A. Incise and drain
    - B. Prescribe antibiotics
    - C. Fenestrate
    - D. **Observe**

63. A 14-year-old female has deep vertical pockets with bone loss on the mesial aspect of all first molars and some drifting of maxillary incisors; however, only minimal inflammation and plaque are present. What is the probable diagnosis?
    - A. Gingivosis
    - B. Periodontitis
    - C. **Periodontosis**
    - D. Osteomyelitis

64. A child aged 7 years comes to the dental clinic for checkup. Upon clinical examination, he reveals a high caries exposure. To achieve a caries reduction, diet modification must be directed toward:
    A. High calcium and vitamin intake
    B. Foods that will buffer the saliva
    C. **"Detergent" foods**
    D. Reduction of carbohydrate intake

65. In a three-and-a-half-year-old male the mandibular second premolars were not evident radiographically. What may be assumed bout these teeth?
    A. Congenitally missing
    B. **May develop late**
    C. Will develop with hypoplastic enamel
    D. Probably extracted

66. While cavity preparation on primary molars in a 5-year-old child the pulp horn that is most likely to be exposed
    A. **Mesiobuccal of first molar**
    B. Distobuccal of first molar
    C. Mesiobuccal of second molar
    D. Distobuccal of second molar

67. While preparing a Class II cavity on the mandibular first molar in a 4-year-old child particular care must be taken while preparing the gingival seat. The reason being
    A. The contact area is broad and flat
    B. The enamel rods incline occlusally
    C. **The tooth has a marked cervical constriction**
    D. The Buccal and lingual tooth surfaces are tapered

68. While preparing an occlusal amalgam preparation in a primary molar in a 3-year-old child what is the recommended relationship of the Buccal and lingual walls?
    A. **Converge at the occlusal**
    B. Diverge at the occlusal
    C. Follow the enamel rods
    D. Parallel to each other

69. A four-year-old child presents with a carious mandibular second primary molar. Caries has reached the pulp, which is vital but hyperemic. What treatment should be performed?
    A. Extraction
    B. Indirect pulp treatment
    C. **Pulpotomy using formocresol**
    D. Pulpotomy using calcium hydroxide

70. A Pulpotomy is performed on a cariously exposed vital mandibular first permanent molar in a seven-year-old child, and calcium hydroxide is placed over the amputation site. What demonstrates a histologically successful treatment?
    A. Eventual Pulpal necrosis
    B. Chronic Pulpal inflammation
    C. **The formation of a dentin bridge slightly below the level of amputation**
    D. The formation of the dentin bridge at a considerable distance from the level of amputation

71. A child age 5 years reports to the dental clinic with pain and swelling associated with lower left first molar which was treated by calcium hydroxide Pulpotomy 1 month back. What is the usual cause of failure of a Pulpotomy that employs the use of calcium hydroxide in a primary molar?
    A. Pulp fibrosis
    B. Pulp necrosis

C. Ankylosis
D. **Internal resorption**

72. An inadvertent mechanical pulp exposure occurs when a cavity on a mandibular first primary molar is prepared. The exposure is less than 1mm in diameter and the treatment was being performed under rubber dam. What treatment should be performed?
    A. **Direct pulp capping**
    B. Indirect pulp capping
    C. Pulpotomy with formocresol
    D. Pulpotomy with calcium hydroxide

73. A child sustains a fracture of a maxillary permanent central incisor. Although the fracture involves only the enamel, there is sufficient loss of tooth tissue for the altered esthetics to be of concern to the parent and child. What treatment at the emergency visit should be performed?
    A. Calcium hydroxide applied to the fracture site and a stainless steel band
    B. Calcium hydroxide applied to the fracture site and a stainless steel crown
    C. **Acid etch composite restoration**
    D. Reduction of tooth for a fabricated acrylic crown

74. A maxillary central incisor in a 10-year-old child gave no response to electrical and thermal pulp tests two days after sustaining a fracture through enamel and dentin. What is the diagnosis of the pulps condition?
    A. Acute hyperemia
    B. Acute necrosis
    C. **No definitive diagnosis of pulp status is possible at this time**
    D. Chronic degeneration

75. A dentist is performing apexification technique on a recently erupted permanent tooth that has been devitalized by trauma? What medicament is generally used?
    A. Zinc oxide eugenol
    B. **Calcium hydroxide alone or with other medicaments**
    C. Formocresol zinc oxide eugenol mixture
    D. Corticosteroids

76. A 9-year-old child is brought to the dental clinic with the chief complaint of a maxillary midline diastema. Which of the following is least likely to cause it
    A. Oral habit
    B. Broadbent phenomenon
    C. High frenal attachment
    D. **High vault palate**

77. A child of 7 years reports to a dental clinic for normal checkup. Which stage of dentition do you expect to see?
    A. Deciduous dentition
    B. Permanent dentition
    C. **First transitional period Mixed dentition**
    D. Intertransitional period Mixed dentition

78. The arch length of a child visiting a dental clinic between the ages of 3 and 18 years will
    A. **Decrease approximately 2mm in the arch**
    B. Decrease approximately 6mm in the arch
    C. Increase approximately 2mm in the arch
    D. Increase approximately 6mm in the arch

79. A two year old reported for an emergency examination of a fractured incisor. What is the most favorable positioning for the patient?
    A. On the dental assistants lap
    B. **On the parents lap**

C. On the dental chair
D. In the papoose board

80. The mothers of which of the following category of children are usually encouraged to remain in the operatory
A. Fearful 6 year old
B. Overprotected 4 year old
C. **Apprehensive 2 year old**
D. Overprotected 6-year-old

81. A 14-year-old female has deep vertical pockets with bone loss on the mesial aspect of all first molars and some drifting of maxillary incisors; however only minimal inflammation and minimal plaque are present. What is the probable diagnosis?
A. Gingivosis
B. Periodontitis
C. **Periodontosis**
D. Osteomylitis

82. A 5 year child reported with a draining fistula in respect to 75. What is the common cause of draining fistulas in gingival tissue in children?
A. Periapical cyst
B. **Chronic periapical abscess**
C. Acute periodontal abscess
D. Acute periapical abscess

83. A 2-year-old child reports with an "eruptive Cyst" in the area of the second molar.
A. **Observe**
B. Incise and drain
C. Excise
D. Prescribe antibiotics

84. A child is diagnosed as having rampant caries. Which of the following teeth and surfaces are characteristically involved
    A. Occlusal surfaces of permanent molars
    B. Proximal surfaces of maxillary incisors
    C. Lingual pits of maxillary molars and incisors and Buccal pits of mandibular molars
    D. **Proximal surfaces of mandibular incisors and cervical areas of any teeth**

85. A 9-year-old child reports with trauma to the upper central incisor with a bluish-grey discoloration. The possible cause of this discoloration is
    A. External resorption
    B. Internal resorption
    C. **Pulpal hemorrhage**
    D. Discolored composite restoration

86. A patient report to the dental clinic and complaints of swollen gingiva since the time he started wearing braces. What is the prognosis for the patient?
    A. **Good: this usually disappears when the bands are removed**
    B. Fair: the gingivitis will probably persist
    C. Poor: periodontitis will probably result in the future
    D. Unpredictable

87. A six monthly dental prophylaxis is prescribed for a child patient achieves which of the following go
    A. Reduce caries incidence by approximately 30 percent
    B. Provide a long term improvement in oral hygiene
    C. **Provide a short term improvement in oral hygiene**
    D. Prevent gingivitis

88. The lactobacillus count of a caries active 16-year-old adolescent is 125,000 lactobacilli per cc of saliva. Based upon the interpretation of this count, what dietary recommendation is indicated
    A. **Temporary elimination of all carbohydrates**
    B. Elimination of between meal consumption of carbohydrates
    C. Increase in dietary consumption of carbohydrates
    D. No dietary modifications are needed

89. During a dental visit, the child may attempt to test the dentist with uncooperative behavior. What should the dentist do?
    A. Dismiss the child and reappoint when better cooperation can be expected
    B. Bribe the child with a gift
    C. **Assert authority and require cooperation**
    D. Engage the child in conversation

90. While restoring a class II in a primary tooth the dentist finds it difficult to adapt the matrix. The probable reason being
    A. Matrices hurt child patient
    B. **Primary teeth converge towards the Occlusal**
    C. Children have small mouths that dislodge the matrix retainers
    D. Children have high gingival attachments

91. The dentist is preparing a deep cavity in a primary molar. Which pulp horn is most likely to be exposed?
    A. **Mesiobuccal of first molar**
    B. Distobuccal of first molar
    C. Mesiobuccal of second molar
    D. Distobuccal of second molar

92. A 4-year-old child presents with a carious mandibular second primary molar. Caries has reached the pulp, which is vital but hyperemic. What treatment should be performed?
    A. Extraction
    B. Pulpotomy using calcium hydroxide
    C. Pulpotomy using formocresol
    D. Indirect pulp treatment

93. An inadvertent mechanical pulp exposure occurs when a cavity on a mandibular first primary molar is prepared. The exposure is small (Less than 1mm) and treatment was being performed under rubber dam. What treatment should be performed?
    A. **Direct pulp capping**
    B. Indirect pulp treatment
    C. Pulpotomy with formocresol
    D. Pulpotomy with calcium hydroxide

94. A child sustains a fracture of a maxillary permanent central incisor. Although the fracture involves only the enamel, there is sufficient loss of tooth tissue for the altered esthetics to be of concern to the parent and child. What treatment at the emergency visit should be performed?
    A. Calcium hydroxide applied to the fracture site and a stainless steel band
    B. Calcium hydroxide applied to the fracture site and a stainless steel crown
    C. **Acid etch composite restoration**
    D. No treatment indicated

95. A maxillary central incisor in a 10-year-old child gave no response to electrical and thermal pulp tests one day after sustaining a fracture through enamel and dentin. What is the diagnosis of the pulp condition?
    A. Acute hyperemia
    B. Acute necrosis

C. **No definitive diagnosis of pulp status is possible**
D. Chronic hyperemia

96. An eight-year-old child who has sustained a fracture of maxillary permanent central incisor in which a large portion of the pulp is exposed presents for treatment three hours after the injury. What emergency treatment of the pulp should be performed?
    A. **Pulpotomy using calcium hydroxide**
    B. Pulpotomy using formocresol
    C. Pulp capping using calcium hydroxide
    D. Pulpectomy and apexification

97. An 8-year-old child reports to the dental clinic with an avulsed 11 within 25 minutes of the trauma. When pulpectomy should be performed
    A. Prior to replantation
    B. Immediately after replantation
    C. Two weeks after replantation
    D. **At a future visit if there is evidence of Pulpal necrosis and root resorption**

98. A child reports with trauma to 21. Upon radiographic evaluation the root shows a fracture. Which of the following areas of root fracture is least conducive to a favorable prognosis
    A. Apical third
    B. Middle third
    C. **Cervical third**
    D. Prognosis is equal in all the cases

99. A dentist is preparing a class I cavity on a primary molar. What is the recommended relationship of the Buccal and lingual walls?
    A. **Converge at the Occlusal**
    B. Parallel to each other
    C. Diverge at the Occlusal
    D. Depends on the extent of the decay

100. When primary molars are prepared for stainless steel crowns, should the depth of reduction of the proximal surfaces be similar to the depth of the Buccal and lingual surfaces?
    A. Reduction of all surfaces is similar for best retention
    B. **Proximal reduction is greater to allow the crown to pass the contact area**
    C. The Buccal surface has the greatest reduction to remove the cervical bulge
    D. All undercuts are uniformly removed so that the steel crown can be seated

101. A 10-year-old child was diagnosed with amelogenesis imperfect with hypoplastic teeth affecting all first permanent molars. What is the treatment of choice for first permanent molars?
    A. Pin retained amalgams
    B. Cast gold crowns
    C. Full upper and lower dentures
    D. **Stainless steel crowns**

102. A 14 year old patient had grossly decayed 36 which need extraction. Which treatment would you prefer to maintain space and restore function
    A. **Removable partial denture**
    B. Implant
    C. No treatment required
    D. Orthodontic treatment

103. How do you prepare class II cavity for amalgam restoration on a tooth 75
    A. **More buccolingual extension**
    B. More gingival
    C. More cervical
    D. More mesiodistal extension

104. A 7 year old child complains of pain while eating food and there is no history of spontaneous pain. On examination, the tooth 85 is decayed, filled with food debris with no sinus or swelling. What is your treatment plan?
    A. **Indirect pulp capping**
    B. Pulpectomy
    C. Extraction
    D. Direct pulp capping

105. While doing pulpotomy for primary tooth, cotton pellet should be
    A. **Dampened with formocresol**
    B. Saturated with formocresol
    C. Left in place for 15 min
    D. Left in place until second visit

106. A parent has come to the clinic with her newborn baby to show the gum pads. There is a tooth like structure on lower anterior region. What is the diagnosis?
    A. Neonatal tooth
    B. **Natal tooth**
    C. Prenatal tooth
    D. Submerged tooth

107. While recording behavior management in case history the following does not include in Frankel behavior rating system
    A. Definitely positive
    B. Definitely negative
    C. **Indifferent**
    D. Positive

108. A 2 ½ year old child has thumb sucking habit. How do you manage?
    A. **Psychological therapy**
    B. Appliance with palatal crib
    C. Ace bandage approach
    D. Dunlop hypothesis

109. In the dental clinic you are using Euphemisms to communicate and manage behavior of the child. What are they?
   A. Fear promoting words
   B. **New words substitutes**
   C. Opposite words
   D. Lisping words

110. A 14 year old child had met with an accident 3 years back. The final diagnosis is Ellis class IV fracture. What are the signs?
   A. Crown enmasse
   B. **Discolored tooth**
   C. Vertical fracture
   D. Root fracture

111. In dental clinics most of the children complains of pain due to
   A. Gingivitis
   B. ANUG and herpes
   C. **Pulpitis and food impaction**
   D. MPDS and aphthous ulcers

112. How do you prepare gingival seat in class II cavity preparation on 65
   A. **Left unbeveled**
   B. Beveled so as to remove caries
   C. Beveled so as to remove unsupported enamel rods
   D. Beveled same as permanent tooth

113. For 2yrs old, what is the quantity of toothpaste you will recommend?
   A. Smear of tooth paste
   B. **Pea-sized amount**
   C. Tooth paste is not recommended
   D. None of the above

114. A tooth has caries involving enamel in 74, you have decided to fill with Glass ionomer cement. Which is correct among following
   A. Is not a Restorative material
   B. Cannot be used as a sealant
   C. **Has improved fluoride release**
   D. Cannot be used as a liner

115. For a 3-year-old child with rampant caries, on first visit what is the procedure performed
   A. Pulp therapy
   B. **Gross excavation and placement of temporary zinc oxide eugenol restoration**
   C. Composite restorations
   D. Extraction

116. According to AAPD, what is the recommended age for first dental examination?
   A. Second year
   B. **Between 6-12 months of age**
   C. When first sign of decay is seen
   D. When child can tolerate dental procedures

117. A 13-year-old patient has come to dental clinic to improve her esthetics. Upon asking history patient has a habit of keeping sweet in her mouth for long time. On examination, she has carious maxillary and mandibular anterior teeth without symptoms. What is the diagnosis?
   A. Nursing bottle caries
   B. Enamel hypoplasia
   C. Tooth fracture
   D. **Rampant caries**

118. How do you calculate Leeway space? It is a difference between sum of the permanent canines and premolars and
    A. **Primary Canines and molars**
    B. Primary Canines + incisors
    C. primary molars
    D. primary incisors

119. For a child having caries in 75, you have decided to do pulpotomy. What is the indication?
    A. Caries involving pulp with intraoral sinus
    B. Mobility
    C. Abscessed tooth
    D. **Spontaneous pain**

120. The most common lesions in anterior teeth seen in pediatric practice is due to
    A. **Nursing bottle caries**
    B. Enamel hypoplasia
    C. Tooth fracture
    D. Peg laterals

121. A 13 year old male patient met with an accident before 30 minutes and complains of missing tooth in upper front tooth region. Parent brought his lost tooth (11) in a container filled with water. What is the treatment?
    A. Take impression for removable partial denture
    B. Checkup and advise medication
    C. **Reimplantation of lost tooth**
    D. Advise to wait and watch

122. A 4 year female patient has caries with no complains of pain in 51 and 61 involving multiple surfaces but without involving pulp. What is your treatment?
    A. Extraction
    B. Temporary restoration
    C. Stainless steel crowns
    D. **Strip crowns**

123. A child of 7-year-old has rampant caries. Which is the wrong statement regarding rampant caries
    A. Rapidly burrowing type of caries
    B. **Mechanism of decay is different**
    C. Can occur suddenly in teeth that were previously sound for many years
    D. Teeth immune to decay are also involved

124. Primate spaces for 3-year-old child in the mandibular arch present
    A. Between permanent mandibular lateral and canine
    B. Between primary mandibular lateral and canine
    C. Between permanent mandibular canine and molar
    D. **Between primary mandibular canine and molar**

125. A seven-year-old boy presented with a painful grossly carious primary molar. Upon examination, tooth 85 is clinically carious, radiographically there is furcation radiolucency and resorption of distal root of 85, half of the premolar is formed, what is your treatment plan
    A. Pulpectomy
    B. Extraction
    C. **Extraction followed by space maintainer**
    D. none of the above

126. A 14-year-old male patient came to the clinic complaining of a localized swelling with a sinus draining pus related to badly decayed 36. The patient has good oral hygiene. Radiographically periapical bone loss is evident. The most probable diagnosis of this case is
   A. Apical periodontitis
   B. Chronic periapical abscess with secondary periodontal involvement
   C. **Asymptomatic irreversible pulpitis with chronic periapical abscess.**
   D. Asymptomatic irreversible pulpitis with asymptomatic apical periodontitis.

127. A 5-year-old patient was diagnosed with rampant caries. On first visit what is the procedure performed
   A. Pulp therapy
   B. **Gross excavation and placement of temporary zinc oxide eugenol restoration**
   C. Composite restorations
   D. none of the above

128. A parent of 7-year-old child complains of swelling of lower lip in her child since two years which is not asymptomatic. There is no history of trauma. What is your diagnosis?
   A. Ranula
   B. Traumatic ulcer
   C. **Mucocele**
   D. Periapical granuloma

129. A patient of 6-year-old has moderate mobility of 74 which is diagnosed as pink tooth. What is the reason for a pink tooth and what is the treatment?
   A. External resorption & Extraction
   B. **Internal resorption & Extraction**
   C. External resorption & Pulpectomy
   D. Internal resorption & Pulpectomy

130. A 10-year-old child attended the clinic with complains of irregular teeth in upper front tooth region. On examination, the upper front teeth are spaced, slightly protruded and there is midline spacing between maxillary incisors. What is your treatment plan?
    A. Orthodontic braces
    B. Composite wire Splinting
    C. **No treatment is required**
    D. Removable partial denture in the space

131. A patient complains of dull and constant pain that lasts 3 days on the left side of the face. The patient noted that the pain increases on positional changes, such as bending over and when jogging. The most likely diagnosis is which of the following
    A. Myocardial infarction
    B. Maxillary sinusitis
    C. Atypical facial pain
    D. **Irreversible pulpitis**

132. After tooth preparation and stainless steel crown placement on 75 in a 6-year-old child, the dentist will take a radiograph. On radiographic examination, the distal aspect of the crown is seating on the occlusal surface of 36. What the dentist supposed to do
    A. Fix the crown in the same position
    B. Take a bigger size crown
    C. **Modify the crown on the distal aspect and fix it**
    D. Modify the crown on the mesial aspect and fix it

133. A seven-year-old boy presented with a painful grossly carious primary incisor. Upon examination, he was found to have multiple other carious teeth requiring full coverage with stainless steel crowns. It is recommended to begin the treatment plan with
    A. Restoration of carious teeth
    B. **Extraction of the grossly carious primary incisor**
    C. Application of fluoride
    D. None of the above

134. A patient of 15-year-old complains of pain in lower left back tooth region since 10 days. On examination, there is no caries except flap covering the erupting molar which is inflamed. What is your treatment plan?
    A. Restoration
    B. **Operculectomy**
    C. Extraction of molar
    D. No treatment required

135. A patient's chief complaint is severe pain from the mandibular right first permanent molar, 46 when eating ice cream and drinking cold water. Clinical examination reveals MOD amalgam restorations in all posterior teeth. The margins appear intact and no cracks or caries is detected. Pulp testing indicates all teeth in the quadrant are responsive to electric pulp testing. Application of cold fails to reproduce the symptoms. Which of the following actions should be taken
    A. The patient should be dismissed and asked to return when the symptoms increase and the pain to cold becomes prolonged.
    B. Initiate root canal treatment by performing a pulpotomy or pulpectomy on tooth 46
    C. Place a rubber dam on individual teeth and apply ice water
    D. **Remove the restoration in tooth 46, place a sedative restoration and prescribe analgesics**

136. While trying the SSC on the prepared tooth, you noticed that there is some resistance with tissue blanching. The reason for this could be
    A. Crown occlusogingival dimension is wrong
    B. Crown mesiodistal dimension is wrong
    C. Tissue caught in margin
    D. **Any of the above could be true**

137. An 11-year-old girl presented with broken upper front tooth due to injury which happened one hour before. Percussion test for the tooth 11 immediately after injury
    A. Gives exact response

B. **Not reliable for diagnosis**
C. Good indication for diagnosis
D. Indicates pulp vitality

138. A 10-year-old child attended the clinic with complains of pain and swelling in upper left back tooth region since 2 days. It was diagnosed as dentoalveolar abscess in relation to 64. After examination, parent slowly revealed the medical history of his child saying that the child is a cardiac patient from birth and is on medication. What is your treatment plan
   A. Extract 64
   B. Medication
   C. Incision and drainage of abscess
   D. **Inform parents to bring consent form from his physician**

139. An 11-year-old child had met with an accident 2 days back. The final diagnosis is Ellis class II fracture. What are the signs?
   A. **Crown fracture**
   B. Discolored tooth
   C. Vertical fracture
   D. Root fracture

140. A 12-year-old child complains of broken upper front tooth which is painful. There is history of trauma one week back. On examination, there is Ellis class III fracture of 11. On soft tissue examination, there is swelling of lower lip. On radiographic examination, there is closed apex of 11 and the broken part of 11 is embedded in lower lip. What is the treatment plan?
   A. RCT for 11, leave the segment in lower lip
   B. Apexogenesis, Surgical removal and reattachment of the segment
   C. **RCT 11, surgical removal and reattachment of the segment**
   D. Apexification of 11

141. A 12-year-old child complains of pain in lower left back tooth region since 2 weeks. On examination, 75 is decayed and having intraoral sinus without mobility. On radiographic examination, radiolucency involving enamel, dentin and pulp. There is absence of premolar tooth bud. Hence, in the absence of premolar tooth bud, the roots of the primary molar will most likely
   A. Resorb at normal site
   B. **Resorb more slowly than normal**
   C. Resorb more rapidly than normal
   D. Show no resorption as the initiator force is absent

142. An infant has come to the clinic with typical bruises, skin lacerations and fractures of bones. Upon asking the parent, parent is unwilling to reveal the history. What is your diagnosis?
   A. Syndromic child
   B. Accidental injury
   C. **Child abuse**
   D. None of the above

143. Disturbances and aberrations in morphodifferentiation stage of tooth development in a 10-year-old child can be seen clinically as
   A. **Peg teeth**
   B. Decrease in number of teeth
   C. Cyst formation
   D. None of the above

144. A 10-year old child presents with mild discomfort in teeth 21 and 22. The teeth were traumatized the day before in a fall from a motorcycle. Clinical examination reveals both teeth are tender to percussion and the crowns are intact. Cold test indicated that the teeth 21 and 22 are not responsive. Treatment plan for such case is
   A. Heat testing for teeth 21, 22
   B. Partial pulpotomy for teeth 21, 22
   C. Root canal treatment for teeth 21, 22

D. **No treatment and follow-up of the patient over the next few weeks**

145. If the child is reluctant to accept the treatment and he appears to be withdrawn. You can give him the Frankl rating scale of

A. One
B. **Two**
C. Three
D. Four

146. While preparing stainless steel crown on 65, the selected crown is not fitting to 65. How do you modify this undersized stainless steel crown for the oversized tooth?

A. Make a cut on the buccal surface of the crown and overlap the margins
B. Make a cut on occlusal surface and spot weld an additional piece of material
C. Make a cut on the lingual surface and overlap the margins
D. **Make a cut on the buccal surface and spot weld an additional piece of material**

147. A 5-year-old patient had grossly decayed 85 which needs extraction. Which treatment would you prefer to maintain space and restore function?

A. Removable partial denture
B. Implant
C. **Pediatric Space maintainer**
D. Orthodontic treatment

148. While doing root canal treatment for 36 in a 12-year-old child, there is a perforation. How do you manage?

A. Extraction
B. Leave the tooth
C. Continue obturation
D. **Seal the perforation and continue RCT**

149. A 7-year male patient has mobility with no complains of pain in 71 and 81. What is your treatment?

   A. Extraction

   B. Temporary restoration

   C. Stainless steel crowns

   D. Wire splinting

150. How do you manage an epileptic child who got seizers on the dental chair during the procedure?

   A. Call the ambulance

   B. Stop the procedure and keep the instruments away

   C. Move away from the child and call the parents

   D. Continue the procedure by using restrainers.

References

AAPD Handbook 4th Edition.

Behavior management in dentistry for children (2nd Ed)(ProQ) G. Z. Wright (Editor)Wiley-Blackwell, 2014.

Clinical cases in pediatric dentistry. A. M. Moursi (Editor) Wiley-Blackwell, 2012.

Clinical problem solving in orthodontics and paediatric dentistry (3rd Ed). D. T. Millett et al.Churchill Livingstone, 2010.

Handbook of clinical techniques in pediatric dentistry(ProQ) J. A. Soxman. Wiley-Blackwell, 2015.

Handbook of Pediatric Dentistry. (Fourth Edition). Edited by:Angus C. Cameron and Richard P. Widmer ISBN: 978-0-7234-3695-9.

Jeffrey AD, Avery DR, McDonald RE. *McDonald and Avery Dentistry for the Child and Adolescent,* 10th Edition.

Kennedy's Pediatric Operative Dentistry. By M. E. J. Curzon (Author), Jessica F. Roberts (Author).

Paediatriccariology (Quintessentials 14)(ProQ) C. Deery Quintessence, 2005.

Paediatric dentistry at a glance(ProQ) A. Cameron et al. Wiley-Blackwell, 2012.

Paediatric Dentistry: 5th Edition by Richard Welbury.

Pediatric Dentistry. Infancy through Adolescence- Jimmy R. Pinkham - 5th.ed. © 2005.

Pediatric Dentistry: A Clinical Approach, 2nd Edition. Goran Koch (Editor), Sven Poulsen(Editor). ISBN: 978-1-118-68719-2.376 pages. May 2013, Wiley-Blackwell.

In: Scenario Based MCQ in Dentistry ISBN: 978-1-53617-298-0
Editors: M. Khursheed Alam et al.

Chapter 10

SCENARIO BASED MCQS IN COMMUNITY DENTISTRY

Nighat Zia Jalbani, Sudhakar Vundavalli and Muhammad Nadeem Baig
Community Dentistry, Preventive Dentistry Department, College of Dentistry, Jouf University, Aljouf, Saudi Arabia

Community Dentistry/Dental Public Health (DPH) is that part of dentistry providing leadership and expertise in population-based dentistry, oral health surveillance, policy development, community-based disease prevention and health promotion, and the maintenance of the dental safety net. DPH and the private practice model of care delivery together bear the responsibility of assuring optimal oral health for all individuals and populations. Public health has been defined in many ways, from "the science and the art of preventing and controlling disease and promoting dental health through organized community efforts" to "a non-clinical specialty of dentistry involved in the assessment of dental health needs and improving the dental health of populations rather than individuals."

This chapter includes questions ranging from basic principles of community dentistry to comprehensive oral health promotion and education concepts along with epidemiological studies to improve the critical thinking of all these concepts by providing the learner with a context to apply knowledge and make decisions. Questions related to pit and fissure sealants, topical and systemic fluorides improve the clinical understanding and importance of these topics. Some of the scenarios leave room for differences in user comprehension and application of knowledge. Advanced epidemiologic scenarios specifically allow different learners to distinguish between similar aspects of observational, analytic study designs and experimental study designs.

The main objective of the Department of Preventive and Community Dentistry is to educate the undergraduate dental students in the:

1) Methods of oral diseases prevention;
2) The applications of Community Dentistry for the promotion of the oral health of the population;
3) The methods of conducting epidemiological studies;
4) In the way behavioral sciences contribute to the understanding and prevention of oral health problems and in the history of Dentistry.

1. A patient comes to you with a buildup of soft deposits within the gingival pockets of his teeth. You also observe the spread of the deposits on marginal gingival tissues. The entire dentition is immensely affected. You are required to score this accumulation of soft deposits according to the criteria established by Silness and Löe in 1964. The following code can be assigned:
   A. 0
   B. 1
   C. 2
   D. 3

2. A new hypoglycemic drug was tried on two groups of diabetic patients in an experimental study, the results of test group came to be more effective in controlling random blood glucose levels as compare to control group using conventional regimen. In this case:
   A. We are rejecting the Null Hypothesis
   B. We are accepting the Null Hypothesis
   C. We are 5% confident that new regimen works
   D. P- value is more than 0.05

3. A clinical case of deep carious lesion along with grade 3 mobility of first left molar with presenting complain of pain on biting and sinus on biting and swelling on buccal aspect of same tooth, indicating need for extraction and prosthetic replacement, this type of case can be categorized as:
   A. Primary prevention
   B. Immediate prevention
   C. Secondary prevention
   D. Tertiary prevention

4. A child patient, approximately 8 years, received fluoride varnish as professionally applied topical fluoride application, specifically to arrest incipient carious lesions, upon follow up after 6 months the child had full developed carious lesions on both lower 1st molars where varnish was applied. The reason for this clinical failure is suspected to arise because:
   A. Child had done vigorous rinsing soon after dental procedure
   B. Lack of use of fluoride toothpaste following procedure
   C. Sticky food use
   D. He missed follow up check ups

5. A study was conducted to check the efficacy of chewing stick (miswak) impregnated with fluoride on group of 50 school children of grade 10. The participants used the stick on right side of mouth for 10 days regularly twice a day and plaque scores were received followed by period of break of 3 days. The plaque scores were repeated after 10 days of use of conventional normal chewing stick (miswak). This kind of study is:
    A. Cross- Over Trials
    B. trials using Split-Mouth Technique
    C. Trials using Passive control
    D. Trials using Positive control

6. 35 patients presented with severe diarrhea and vomiting after having dinner in a local restaurant, 50 students were served dinner out of that 35 suffered from acute episode of gastritis following eating of undercooked meat. The sudden occurrence of this outbreak of specific illness from a single source, in a group of students is called:
    A. Pandemic
    B. Endemic
    C. Epidemic
    D. Emergency

7. In 1945 there were 1,000 women who worked in a factory painting radium dials on watches. The incidence of bone cancer in these women up to 1975 was compared with that of 1,000 women who worked as telephone operators in 1975. Twenty of the radium dial painters and four of the telephone operators developed bone cancer between 1945 and 1975. This study is an example of a:
    A. Experimental study
    B. Case-control study
    C. Clinical trial
    D. Cohort study

8. The mean birth weight of first-born infants of 23 women who smoked more than one pack of cigarettes per day during pregnancy was 200 g lower than those of the first-born infants of 16 women who never smoked, the difference was statistically significant at the 5% level (P<0,05). This means which of the following?
   A. The difference observed between mean birth weights was too large to have occurred by chance alone
   B. The difference observed between mean birth weights could have been easily occurred by chance alone
   C. The number of patients studied was not sufficient to achieve a conclusive result
   D. Smoking during pregnancy does not influence fetal growth

9. In a well-designed clinical trial of treatment of ovarian cancer, remission rate at one year is similar for a new drug and usual care, The P-value is 0.4. This means that:
   A. Both treatments are effective
   B. Neither treatment is effective
   C. The statistical power of this study is 60%
   D. It is not possible to decide on whether one treatment is better than the other using this information alone

10. Investigators are studying employees at a bus company to test their hypothesis that occupational stress causes high blood pressure. Two major groups of employees are of interest: bus drivers and office workers with same salary scale. Age, sex, ethnicity and length of employment were kept common for both groups of workers. The mean blood pressure of the bus drivers is found to be higher than office workers and investigators concluded that stress causes high blood pressure. The type of study this would be:
   A. Experimental
   B. Observational
   C. Case series
   D. Hypothetical case testing

11. One hundred Persons with Hepatitis A and 100 healthy neighbors were questioned regarding their history of eating raw clams or oysters in the preceding 3 months: if this study design is observational in nature what is sub type of this:
    A. cohort
    B. case- control
    C. Retrospective cohort
    D. Prospective cohort

12. In one of developing countries the death of infants were recorded to be 6.3 per 1000 live births in 2000, in 2005 the death of infants reduced to 5.7 per 1000 live births. From this example we can calculate:
    A. Proportion
    B. Incidence
    C. Simple count number of infant deaths
    D. Rate

13. In a government hospital a team of highly professional Public Health professionals delivered a workshop for nursing staff. The training of nursing staff was upgraded in terms of giving more preventive care than curative based strategies. This type of workshop and training aims to implement and improve:
    A. Health education among staff
    B. Health promotion and health education
    C. Re-orient health services
    D. Improving personal professional skills

14. Number of dental students planned to visit government schools of Sakaka Al Jouf to improve knowledge of dental health education regarding daily oral hygiene activities among school teachers, parents and school children. Pamphlets, posters and electronic media prints were distributed randomly. This is called:
    A. Formal health education
    B. Informal health education

C. Planned school visit
D. Health promotion

15. A research study regarding association between severity of periodontal disease among heavy and chain smokers was conducted. After preliminary planning was completed, 15 numbers of smokers were initially orally examined and results were compared and modifications were made accordingly. This type of preliminary testing is called:
    A. Cross-sectional study
    B. One-time study
    C. Pilot study
    D. Reverse cohort

16. Of the following, the true statement is:
    A. Fluoridation has its greatest effect in the lower social groups and appeared to remove inter-social class differences in dental caries experience
    B. The first city to fluoridate in UK was East London
    C. Fluoride has been found to have no beneficial effect for the prevention of root caries
    D. Fluoride is being used regularly and effectively in treating osteoporosis

17. Communities without fluoridation also benefit from foods and drinks processed in communities with fluoridation and sold or used in communities without fluoridation. This effect is called:
    A. Dilution effect
    B. Dispersion effect
    C. Diffusion effect
    D. Submissive effect

18. A child aged 6 – 16-year-old consumes drinking water with the fluoride concentration of more than 0.6 ppm. The fluoride supplement dosage should be
    A. 0 mg
    B. 0.25 mg
    C. 0.50 mg
    D. 1 mg

19. The cost of salt fluoridation is higher than water fluoridation. Salt fluoridation reaches a wide population irrespective of geographic location and economy.
    A. 1st statement is true, 2nd statement is false
    B. 1st statement is false, 2nd statement is true
    C. Both the statements are true
    D. Both the statements are false

20. If the concentration of fluoride in the water is 0.5PPM, and the age of the child is 4 years, then the fluoride supplement to given to the child is:
    A. 0 mg
    B. 0.25 mg
    C. 0.50 mg
    D. mg

21. Among the following predictors for caries in a population, the most powerful factor is:
    A. Mutans streptococci and lactobacillus colonies count
    B. History of frequent sugar intake
    C. No fluoride exposure
    D. Past caries prevalence

22. All is true regarding the absorption of fluoride, *except*
    A. Fluoride ingested with a glass of milk, there is 100% absorption
    B. Absorption of fluoride is influenced by degree of ionization of the compounds
    C. Calcium increases the absorption of fluoride considerably
    D. Fluoride absorption is different for different species

23. The concentration of fluoride is negligible in soft tissues, because:
    A. The cells do not have microvilli to absorb fluoride
    B. There are no hydroxyl ions or any other alike negative ion to be replaced
    C. The pH of soft tissue is not acidic to form hydrofluoric acid
    D. All of the above

24. Recommended average daily intake of fluoride from all sources. Combined for adults &child is:
    A. 0.2 to 1.2mg & 0 – 0.5mg
    B. 1.2 to 2.2 mg & 0.5 – 1.0mg
    C. 2.2 to 3.2 mg & 1.0 – 1.2mg
    D. 3.2 to 4.2 mg & 1.8mg

25. Everything about the concentration of fluoride in bone is true, *except*
    A. Bones of mature animals take up less fluoride than the young ones
    B. Cancellous bones incorporate more fluoride than Compact bones
    C. Cortical bone incorporates more fluoride than periosteal bone
    D. There is initial rapid fluoride uptake followed by slow uptake.

26. Everything about the concentration of fluoride in the teeth is true, *except*
    - A. Fluoride concentration in enamel is highest in the cervical region in the old age
    - B. Fluoride concentration in dentin is highest in the pulpal region
    - **C. Fluoride concentration in enamel surface reduces considerably with age**
    - D. Fluoride concentration in cementum is highest in the surface

27. All is true about the influence of age on fluoride uptake, *except*
    - A. The concentration of fluoride in enamel increases with age in the cervical areas
    - **B. The concentration of fluoride in enamel increases with age in the incisal areas**
    - C. The concentration of fluoride increases steadily in dentin with age
    - D. The concentration of fluoride increases with age in the cementum

28. As age increases, the concentration of fluoride near DEJ in dentin increases. The concentration of fluoride in dentin is highest near DEJ.
    - A. 1st statement is true; 2nd statement is false.
    - B. 1st statement is false, 2nd statement is true
    - C. Both the statements are true
    - **D. Both the statements are false**

29. The fluoride content on the outer surface of enamel of central incisors is more than lateral incisors. As age advances, the outer surface of enamel incorporates more fluoride on the gingival third of the teeth.
    - A. 1st statement is true; 2nd statement is false.
    - **B. 1st statement is false, 2nd statement is true**
    - C. Both the statements are true
    - D. Both the statements are false

30. A 5-year old child consumes 80 mg F with milk accidentally. The mode of treatment for this child is:
    A. No treatment required
    B. Give calcium orally
    C. Induce vomiting
    D. Give calcium + induce vomiting

31. Students begin arriving at Health services with severe cough that includes bloody phlegm. The physicians and nurses interview some of the early cases and find out that many of them mention attending a party at which a new (to them) batch of marijuana was smoked. A prime source of epidemiological hypotheses is 'clinical hunches', of which this is an example – the clinicians develop the hunch that a specific batch of marijuana may be responsible for this previously unrecognized respiratory illness. What is the name of the research design from which this hunch was derived?
    A. Case control
    B. Cohort (Retrospective)
    C. Cohort (Prospective)
    D. Case series

32. The key factor in conducting ethical research is:
    A. Informed consent
    B. Beneficence
    C. Justice
    D. Respect for persons

33. Confidentiality means that:
    A. The identity of the participant is not recorded
    B. The principal investigator and staff have guaranteed that identifying information will not be revealed

C. The principal investigator does not know the identity of the participants
D. The funding agency does not know the identity of the participants.

34. Which type of study assesses the efficacy of the treatment intervention in a controlled, standardized, and highly monitored setting and usually among highly selected samples of patients?
A. Randomized controlled trial
B. Case series
C. Sensitivity analysis
D. Cost benefit analysis

35. In order to receive funding from the National Institutes of Health for funding of studies in developing countries, the principal investigator must receive approval from an ethics committee that:
A. Includes epidemiologists
B. Includes clergy from the local religions
C. Has received a federal-wide assurance
D. Has been approved by the Minister of Health of the country

36. Placebos may be used in clinical trials when:
A. The alternative treatment is very expensive
B. There is no reasonably available alternative treatment
C. The standard treatment is associated with a risk of adverse side effects
D. a and c above

37. An environmental, behavioral, or biological factor that directly increases the probability of occurrence of a disease is called
A. Risk factor
B. Risk Indicator
C. Demographic risk factor
D. Risk marker

38. Scale in which the conditions in some order of severity but the categories do not have a mathematical relationship with one another is known as
    - A. Nominal scale
    - **B. Ordinal scale**
    - C. Interval scale
    - D. Ratio scale

39. A new drug was introduced in some of patients to assess its usefulness compared with the old one. Neither patients nor clinicians who evaluated patients for effect under consideration in this clinical trial knew individual treatment assignments. This method of assignment is known as:
    - **A. Single blinding**
    - B. Double blinding
    - C. Triple blinding
    - D. Randomization

40. If a manufacturer wants to test fluoride toothpaste with a stronger formulation than the standard one, this type of trial should be using:
    - A. Historical controls
    - B. Self-controls
    - C. Passive controls
    - **D. Positive controls**

41. The data taken from the population in which samples are taken from different age groups, sex groups and income groups are known as:
    - A. Cluster sampling
    - B. Multistage sampling
    - **C. Stratified sampling**
    - D. Systematic sampling

42. When drug is evaluated for its usefulness in controlled conditions, it is termed as trial signifying:
    - **A. Efficacy**
    - B. Effect modification
    - C. Effectiveness
    - D. Efficiency

43. Of a specific disease the number of new cases occurring in a defined population during a specified period of time is known as:
    - A. Prevalence
    - B. Distribution
    - **C. Incidence**
    - D. Point prevalence

44. The health educator offering weight control and exercise programs is an example of
    - A. information dissemination
    - B. health risk appraisal and wellness assessment
    - **C. lifestyle and behavior change**
    - C. environmental control program

45. Distributing stress management pamphlets and presenting a poster exhibit at a health fair is an example of
    - **A. information dissemination**
    - B. health risk appraisal and wellness assessment
    - C. lifestyle and behavior change
    - D. environmental control program

46. A National Health survey in 2015 revealed burden of 3000 people cases of diabetic people in population of 10,000, in 2016 the number of diabetic people exceeded to 3500. What kind of measure we can calculate from this scenario?
    - A. Count
    - B. Incidence only

C. Prevalence only

D. Incidence and prevalence both

47. The statement "Dental health education programs can temporarily improve knowledge and oral hygiene but have not demonstrated any direct effect on caries experience":

    A. Is one of the principles of oral health education that has emerged from literature

    B. Is one of the assumed misunderstandings emerged from past experience of studies?

    C. Is one of the facts about oral health promotion?

    D. Is proven statement summarized by dental professionals?

48. The approach in which health services needed by the people are provided at their door steps on the assumption that people would use them to improve their own health is:

    A. Regulatory approach

    B. Service approach

    C. Health education approach

    D. Primary health care approach

49. The approach of health education in which there is governmental intervention, direct/indirect, designed to alter human behavior is:

    A. Regulatory approach

    B. Service approach

    C. Health education approach

    D. Primary health care approach

50. The types of discussion in which all the members participate and arrive at a decision on that particular topic is called:

    A. Panel discussion

    B. Group discussion

    C. Symposium

    D. Workshop

51. While planning for a clinical trial for finding out the effect of a particular mouth wash on human subjects, which kind of study design will be able to give best results:
    - **A. Randomized controlled trial with double blinding**
    - B. Randomized controlled trial with no blinding
    - C. Non-randomized controlled trial
    - D. Randomized controlled trial with single blinding

52. A clinical trial was done to test efficacy of a Fluoride tooth paste on a group of subjects. In this trial neither participants not the examiners were aware of the group allocation. This type of study is usually called:
    - A. Single blind study
    - **B. Double blind study**
    - C. Triple blind study
    - D. Longitudinal study

53. A new treatment regimen was tried on test group in an experimental study, the results of test group are not different from control group who is using conventional regimen:
    - A. We are rejecting the Null Hypothesis
    - **B. We are accepting the Null Hypothesis**
    - C. We are 95% confident that new regimen works
    - D. The chance of accepting the null hypothesis is only 5% (P=less than 0.05)

54. The scale of measuring oral diseases in which there is neither mathematical relationship nor an order among the categories is:
    - A. Nominal scale
    - **B. Interval scale**
    - **C.** Ordinal scale
    - D. Ratio scale

55. Suppose you have 2 sets of data for measuring pocket depth of first molar: one in mm and the other in cm. The best method to compare the dispersion of data for the two groups is:
    A. Standard deviation
    B. Range
    C. Coefficient of variation
    D. Mean

56. A clinical trial using Vitamin C and placebo tablets was conducted to find out whether Vitamin C prevents gingivitis or not. The most appropriate statistical test to test the Null Hypothesis in this case is:
    A. Chi-square
    B. t-test
    C. z-test
    D. f-test

57. A group of 200 students were tested on their presentation skills before undertaking a presentation development session, after which they were tested again. Which statistical test is most relevant to determining whether the presentation development course had a significant effect?
    A. Independent t test
    B. Wilcoxon
    C. Mann-Whitney
    D. Paired sample t-test

58. The incidence of oral cancer per one lakh population in an area is reported as 230, 240, 300, 200, 20, 240, 310 and 800.The best value (mean or median or mode) to give the idea about the incidence of oral cancer is:
    A. Arithmetic Mean
    B. Geometric mean
    C. Median
    D. Mode

59. Most commonly used measure of central dispersion is:

    A. Mean
    B. Inter quartile range
    C. Standard deviation
    D. Coefficient of variance

60. Two variables can be plotted and compared in:

    A. Pie chart
    B. Histogram
    C. **Scatter diagram**
    D. Bar diagram

61. Calculate athematic mean for the following set of values 12, 10, 8, 6, 16 and 20.

    A. 14
    B. 12
    C. 16
    D. 11

62. Identify Median for the following set of values: 12, 10, 8, 6,16, 15 and 16.

    A. 16
    B. 10
    C. 12
    D. 11

63. Among the following methods of data presentation, the one which suits best for laymen or people who can't understand technical terms?

    A. Line diagram
    B. Pictogram
    C. Scatter Diagram
    D. Frequency polygon

64. Age of the children and number of teeth erupted were assessed in a descriptive study among school children of Sakaka. Which measure of central dispersion is appropriate in this scenario?
    A. Range
    B. Mean deviation
    C. Standard deviation
    D. Coefficient of Variance

65. In a normal distribution curve, Mean±2SD includes
    A. 95% of all observations
    B. 97% of all observations
    C. 68% of all observation
    D. 99% of all observation

66. Number of teeth present in oral cavity is an example for
    A. Qualitative data
    B. Discrete data
    C. Continuous data
    D. Nominal data

67. The average anatomical length of the crown of maxillary canines was 9.61 mm, which is an example for
    A. Continuous data
    B. Discrete data
    C. Qualitative data
    D. Ordinal data

68. The best measure of central tendency for ordinal data
    A. Mean
    B. Geometric mean
    C. Standard deviation
    D. Median

69. The names of the bones like Mandible, maxilla, femur, etc. are examples for
    A. Quantitative data
    B. Nominal data
    C. Ordinal data
    D. Continuous data

70. Diabetes mellitus is considered as one of the risk factor for periodontal disease. In the following table cases are the people who have periodontal disease and controls are healthy group. Calculate the odds ratio between diabetes and periodontal disease using the table below.

	Controls (Healthy)	Cases (Periodontal disease)
Diabetics	**3**	**7**
Non-Diabetics	**8**	**4**
Total	**11**	**11**

    A. 5.2
    B. 4.6
    C. 3.4
    D. 6

71. Various grades of dental fluorosis like normal, very mild, mild, moderate and severe is an example of?
    A. Quantitative data
    B. Nominal data
    C. Ordinal data
    D. Continuous data

72. A research was conducted to assess the Blood pressure levels in males and females. Which statistical test is appropriate for comparison above factors?
    A. Students 't' test/Unpaired 't" test
    B. Paired 't' test

C. Chi-square test
D. Pearson's correlation

73. The anxiety level of 25 randomly selected students was measured by taking their blood pressure before and after an examination. Suppose the blood pressure scores were normally distributed in the study population. The most appropriate statistical test that can be used in this scenario is?
The following table shows Information contained in five patient charts from a periodontal office is summarized in the following. Three observations, sex, age, and pocket depth, were made for each of the five patients.

Patient No	Gender	Age	Pocket Depth
1	M	38	3.5
2	F	45	4
3	M	60	5
4	F	44	4
5	M	62	6.5
6	F	53	4

A. Independent sample t-test
B. Chi-square test
C. Paired t-test
D. Kappa test

74. The Pocket depth as a variable is considered as:
A. Qualitative Nominal
B. Qualitative Ordinal
C. Quantitative discrete
D. Quantitative Continuous

75. The mean pocket depth for males is

A. 3.5

B. 4

C. 5

D. 6.5

76. The Standard deviation (SD) for Females pocket depth is:

A. No SD

B. 0

C. 1

D. 4

77. The data for this group of data is:

A. Unimodal data

B. Bimodal data

C. Trimodal data

D. No mode

78. If a class test was generally very easy for most of the students with only a few getting very low scores, then the distribution of scores would be:

A. Positively skewed

B. Negatively skewed

C. Not skewed at all

D. Normal

79. When a group of study subjects is classified in three categories according to the severity of gingivitis as mild, moderate and severe, the scale of measurement used is:

A. Interval scale

B. Ratio scale

C. Nominal scale

D. Ordinal scale

80. The branch of biostatistics that deals with generalization of the results obtained from a sample to the study population is:
    A. Summative
    B. Inferential
    C. Analytic
    D. Descriptive

81. Use of type A dentifrice and type B dentifrice will show no difference in caries reduction. This statement is an example of:
    A. Null hypothesis
    B. Alternative hypothesis
    C. Type I error
    D. Type II error

82. To evaluate the statistical significance of the difference between two sample means, we should use:
    A. Chi-square test
    B. One sample t-test
    C. Independent sample t-test
    D. Paired sample t-test

83. Dental flossing is one of the oral hygiene measures to combat caries-inducing microorganisms at home by the individual patient. When flossing should be started?
    A. At the age of 5 years old
    B. At the age of 4 years old
    C. At the age of 3 years old
    D. At the age of 6 years old

84. One of following concentration of fluoride is recommended in school water fluoridation when community water supply is not fluoridated:
    A. 4.5 ppm
    B. 3.5 ppm
    C. 2.5 ppm
    D. 1.5 ppm

85. While planning for a clinical trial for finding out the effect of a particular mouth wash on human subjects, which kind of study design will be able to give best results:
    A. Randomized controlled trial with double blinding
    B. Randomized controlled trial with no blinding
    C. Non-randomized controlled trial
    D. Randomized controlled trial with single blinding

86. A clinical trial was done to test efficacy of a Fluoride tooth paste on a group of subjects. In this trial neither participants not the examiners were aware of the group allocation. This type of study is usually called:
    A. Single blind study
    B. Double blind study
    C. Triple blind study
    D. Longitudinal study

87. Routine data collected on hospitalised patients and in population censuses and health surveys is type of:
    A. Experimental studies
    B. Analytic study designs
    C. Cross-sectional studies
    D. Ecological studies

88. Clinical trial used for testing agents that prevent reversible conditions like gingivitis or calculus is called:
    A. Cross-Over Trials
    B. trials using Split-Mouth Technique
    C. Trials using Passive control
    D. Trials using Positive control

89. A new treatment regimen was tried on test group in an experimental study, the results of test group are not different from control group who is using conventional regimen:
    A. We are rejecting the Null Hypothesis
    B. We are accepting the Null Hypothesis
    C. We are 95% confident that new regimen works
    D. The chance of accepting the null hypothesis is only 5% (P=less than 0.05)

90. A survey that incorporates sufficient examination sets to cover all important subgroups of the population and at least 3 of the age groups/index ages is:
    A. Pilot survey
    B. Need based assessment survey
    C. National pathfinder survey
    D. Pathfinder survey

91. Among the index age groups recommended by WHO, the index age chosen for caries for international comparisons and monitoring of disease trends is:
    A. 12-year-old
    B. 15-year-old
    C. 35-44-year-old
    D. 65-74-year-old

92. The relationship between reliability and validity of a question is such that:

    A. A valid question must be reliable

    B. A reliable question is also valid

    C. Validity and reliability have no relation

    D. Validity is dependent upon reliability

93. Forensic dentistry involves the study of teeth with the intention of providing facts to be used as evidence in court. What is another name for this field of study?

    A. forensic entomology

    B. forensic odontology

    C. forensic palynology

    D. forensic entomology

94. When skeletons are found, the teeth are an important source of information. In such cases, which of the following statements is the most accurate?

    A. Teeth can indicate a person's occupation

    B. Teeth can indicate a person's age

    C. Teeth can indicate a person's ethnic background

    D. All three statements are true

95. Bite marks appear as circular or oval patterned injury consisting of two opposing U-shaped arches, one type is Partial bite where part of the tissue has been torn away.

    A. Both are incorrect

    B. Both statements are correct

    C. First one is incorrect while the second is correct

    D. First one is correct while the second incorrect

96. The forensic dentist compares ___________ with postmortem records to determine if there is a positive match.
   A. Ante mortem
   B. A smiling photograph
   C. Shovel-shaped incisors
   D. the AFBO scale

97. When palatal Rugae measure 2-3mm in a straight line from medial to lateral direction it should be categorized as:
   A. Negligible rugae
   B. Secondary rugae
   C. Primary Rugae
   D. Fragmentary rugae

98. The pulp cavity of molars is wide and deep while the roots are fused and bent "Taurodontism" are characteristic features for:
   A. Negroid race
   B. South African
   C. Caucasoid race
   D. Mongoloid race

99. All of the following are characteristic to the mandible during adulthood *except*
   A. Ramus forms an obtuse angle with the body
   B. Body is thick and long
   C. Condyles are elongated and project above the coronoid
   D. Mental foramen is midway between upper and lower margins

100. The most important specialty of today's forensic sciences is:
   A. Ballistics.
   B. DNA profiling
   C. Fingers prints analysis
   D. Forensic Toxicology

References

Burt A. B., Eklund S. A. Dentistry, *Dental Practice and the Community*. 6th Ed 2005, W. B.

Hiremath S. S. *Textbook of Preventive and Community Dentis*try, 2nd Edition,2016.

Katz, David L., Elmore, Joann G., Wild, Dorothea M. G. and Lucan, Sean C. 10, *Jekel's Epidemiology, Biostatistics, Preventive Medicine, and Public Health*, 4th edition, 119-133. Copyright © 2014, 2007, 2001, 1996 by Saunders, an imprint of Elsevier Inc.

Park Textbook of Preventive and Social Medicine PDF Book. 2015, Part of the 23rd Edition series. Saunders Company.

In: Scenario Based MCQ in Dentistry ISBN: 978-1-53617-298-0
Editors: M. Khursheed Alam et al.

Chapter 11

SCENARIO BASED MCQS IN DENTAL ANATOMY

Krishna A. Rao[1], MDS,
Manay Srinivas Munisekhar[2], MDS
and Farahnaz Muddebihal[2], MDS
[1]Oral Pathology, Preventive Dentistry Department,
College of Dentistry, Jouf University, Aljouf, Saudi Arabia
[2]Preventive Dentistry Department,
College of Dentistry, Jouf University, Aljouf, Saudi Arabia

Dental anatomy, also known as Dental morphology, is a specialized branch of dentistry that discusses tooth morphology along with its applications & terminologies related to the practice of dentistry. It focusses on the most important details of tooth morphology. It also has an overview of various geometrical outlines, the physiological tooth formation protecting the periodontium, the description of pulp cavities in the permanent teeth, as well as shedding light on the arrangement of permanent teeth and a brief idea about occlusion. It also deals with the various tooth notation systems, dentition periods, as well as the chronology and sequence of eruption of both dentitions.

Great care has been taken to confirm the accuracy of the information presented and the generally described terminologies. The authors, along with the contributors, believe this is a sincere attempt to refresh the knowledge of dental anatomy taught at the preliminary stage of undergraduate study. Solving these questions will help students in refreshing their basic understanding of the subject, which becomes highly essential while answering dental anatomy questions in the competitive exams they take up at various levels. However, students are advised to go through the reference textbooks mentioned to become more competent and confident while attempting the exams.

1. According to FDI system, the maxillary right first premolar is represented as:
    A. 24
    B. 14
    C. 20
    D. 28

2. Which of the following statements is not true regarding a 'Tubercle'
    A. It is a small elevation on some portion of the crown
    B. It represents a lobe
    C. It is deviation from normal
    D. It is formed only of enamel

3. Identify the TRUE statement regarding the Maxillary Permanent Central Incisors
    A. Mesial contact area is more cervical than the distal contact area
    B. The crown completion takes place around 7-8 years
    C. The labio-lingual dimension is greater than mesio-distal dimension
    D. Incisal third appears thicker distally as compared to that seen from the mesial aspect

4. All the following statements regarding Maxillary Permanent Canine are TRUE *except*
   A. The mesial contact areais at junction of incisal and middle $1/3^{rd}$
   B. The mesial slope of the cuspis shorter than the distal slope
   C. The cusp tip when viewed from the proximal aspects is centralized on the long axis or inclined labially
   D. Crown of maxillary canine is longer and narrower than mandibular canine

5. Maxillary premolars has some characteristics common to all posterior teeth, they are
   A. Larger crown
   B. Narrowcontact area
   C. Great buccolingual dimension than the mesiodistal
   D. Morecurvature of cervical line mesially and distally

6. While building the crown of Mandibular 1st premolar, the unique characteristic of mandibular 1st premolar has to be retained by creating
   A. Distal marginal ridge occlusal to Mesial marginal ridge
   B. Mesial marginal ridge occlusal to Distal marginal ridge
   C. Distal marginal ridge cervical to Mesial marginal ridge
   D. Both Distal and Mesial marginal ridges at the same level

7. All the following statements are TRUE regarding Mandibular 2nd premolar *except*
   A. The lingual cusps are shorter than the buccal cusps and are more pointed
   B. There is no lingual convergence in the three-cusp type variant
   C. Mesiolingual cusp is longer and larger than the distolingual cusp
   D. The lingual developmental groove demarcates the mesiolingual from distolingual cusp

8. While restoring the occlusal aspect of Maxillary Permanent 1st molar, the oblique ridge should be carved between
   A. Mesiolingual triangular ridge and distobuccal distal ridge
   B. Triangular ridges of distobuccal and distolingual cusps
   C. Mesiolingual distal ridge and distobuccal triangular ridge
   D. Triangular ridges of mesiobuccal and distolingual cusps

9. During fabrication of crown of Maxillary Permanent 1st molar, when viewed from the occlusal aspect, the obtuse angles should be maintained for
   A. Mesiobuccal and distolingual line angles
   B. Mesiolingual and distobuccal line angles
   C. Mesiobuccal and distobuccal line angles
   D. Mesiolingual and distolingual line angles

10. During restoration of the Class I cavity on the occlusal aspect of Maxillary Permanent 1st molar, the developmental groove of oblique ridge on the occlusal aspect of Maxillary Permanent First Molar should be carved in the form of
    A. Central groove
    B. Buccal groove.
    C. Transverse groove
    D. Lingual groove

11. While fabricating the crown of Mandibular Permanent 1st molar, which of the following instruction should be given to the dental technician
    A. To create a wider and longer mesiolingual cusp than the distolingual cusp
    B. To create wider and longer mesiobuccal cusp than the distobuccal and distal cusps
    C. To make the mesiobuccal and distobuccal cusps more sharper and conical
    D. To make the crown wider buccolingually than mesiodistally

12. During fabrication of a complete denture, in the maximum intercuspal position, which two teeth occlude with the maxillary 1st premolar
    - **A. Mandibular first & second premolars**
    - B. Mandibular canine & first premolar
    - C. Mandibular second premolar & first molar
    - D. Mandibular canine & mandibular second premolar

13. What is the clinical attachment loss of a tooth with +2 mm of gingival recession & a 4 mm pocket
    - A. + 2 mm
    - B. 6 mm
    - C. 2 mm
    - **D. + 6 mm**

14. A 3 year old boy reported to a dental clinic with pain in the lower left side of jaw. On intraoral examination, the posterior tooth showed deep carious lesion. Identify the affected tooth number?
    - **A. 75**
    - B. 85
    - C. 45
    - D. 35

15. Identify which tooth of lower jaw contains central developmental groove in form of H and U?
    - A. Mandibular first premolar
    - B. Maxillary first premolar
    - **C. Mandibular second premolar**
    - D. Maxillary second premolar

16. If there is loss of posterior teeth in the lower jaw, this could lead to elongation of upper posterior teeth and migration of neighboring lower teeth to fill the space. This could further lead to disturbance in
    A. Speech
    B. Centric occlusion
    C. Swallowing
    D. Eating

17. Tooth number 16 followed by tooth number 46 are considered as key of occlusion for which of the following reasons?
    A. They are second permanent teeth to develop in oral cavity
    B. They are the smallest teeth in the dental arch
    C. Their positions are guided by presence of deciduous molars preceding them
    D. Their eruption is disturbed as they have no predecessor

18. A 2 year old girl reported with pain and swelling in upper right second molar. What could be the FDI tooth number,
    A. 55
    B. 65
    C. 85
    D. 75

19. Identify in which of the following teeth a developmental groove crosses the mesial marginal ridge and forms a mesial marginal developmental groove.
    A. Mandibular 1st premolar
    B. Mandibular 2nd premolar
    C. Maxillary 1st premolar
    D. Maxillary 2nd premolar

20. Identify on which cusp does the fifth cusp of maxillary permanent first molar appear?
    A. Mesiobuccal cusp
    B. Distobuccal cusp
    C. Mesiolingual cusp
    D. Distolingual cusp

21. A 2 year old boy complains of dental caries in upper right second molar. Identify to which permanent teeth does this upper right second molar resemble?
    A. Maxillary Permanent first premolar
    B. Maxillary Permanent second premolar
    C. Maxillary Permanent second molar
    D. Maxillary Permanent first molar

22. Canine fossa is seen in
    A. Maxillary permanent canine
    B. Mandibular permanent canine
    C. Maxillary first premolar
    D. Mandibular first premolar

23. The maxillary first premolar differs from the other premolars
    A. In the number of buccal cusps
    B. Geometric outline of the crown from the buccal aspect
    C. Geometric outline of the crown from the lingual aspect
    D. In the mesial and distal slopes of the buccal cusp

24. Which of the following premolars has the smallest lingual cusp?
    A. Maxillary second premolar
    B. Mandibular first premolar
    C. Mandibular second premolar
    D. Maxillary first premolar

25. Which of the following premolars has a central fossa?
    A. Mandibular second premolar
    B. Maxillary second premolar
    C. Mandibuar first premolar
    D. Maxillary first premolar

26. Cusp of Carabelli is seen in
    A. Maxillary permanent second molar
    B. Mandibular permanent first molar
    C. Maxillary deciduous first molar
    D. Maxillary deciduous second molar

27. Which of the following teeth shows buccal convergence?
    A. Maxillary permanent central incisor
    B. Maxillary permanent first molar
    C. Mandibular permanent central incisor
    D. Mandibular permanent first molar

28. Which of the following has the least contribution in the health of the interdental papilla?
    A. Proximal contact points
    B. Embrasures
    C. Cervical ridge
    D. Interproximal spaces

29. In an extracted upper first molar, buccal curvature is noted in
    A. Mesiobuccal canal
    B. Distobuccal canal
    C. Palatal canal
    D. Cusp of Carabelli

30. When a child reaches nine years of age, mandibular first permanent molar has its distal contact with which of the following teeth?
    A. First premolar
    B. No distal contact
    C. Deciduous Second molar
    D. Permanent Second molar

31. When upper and lower teeth of a 24 year old male are in maximum intercuspation, it is referred as
    A. Centric occlusion
    B. Centric bite
    C. Centric position
    D. Centric relation

32. Identify the last succedaneous tooth to erupt in oral cavity?
    A. Maxillary canine
    B. Mandibular canine
    C. Maxillary third molar
    D. Mandibular third molar

33. Steepest cusp inclination is noted in which of the permanent tooth?
    A. Maxillary 1st premolar
    B. Maxillary 2nd premolar
    C. Mandibular 1st premolar
    D. Mandibular 2nd premolar

34. Identify which of the following sequence of eruption for maxillary permanent tooth is correct?
    A. 6, 1, 2, 4, 3, 5, 7, 8
    B. 6, 1, 2, 3, 4, 5, 7, 8
    C. 6, 1, 2, 3, 4, 5, 8, 7
    D. 6, 1, 3, 2, 4, 7, 5, 8

35. A 2 year old boy reported with dental caries in lower right second molar. What could be the FDI tooth number
    A. 55
    B. 65
    C. 85
    D. 75

References

Dubrel. *Oral Anatomy*, 8th Edition.

Head, Neck and Dental Anatomy, Marjorie J. Short, Deborah Levin Goldstein, 4th Edition, Printed in United States of America.

Major M. Ash. Wheeler's Dental Anatomy, *Physiology and amp.; Occlusion,* 9 th Edition. Saunders Company, 2010.

Scheid. *Woelfel's Dental Anatomy*, 8th Edition.

In: Scenario Based MCQ in Dentistry ISBN: 978-1-53617-298-0
Editors: M. Khursheed Alam et al.

Chapter 12

SCENARIO BASED MCQS IN ORAL BIOLOGY

Manay Srinivas Munisekhar, MDS, Farahnaz Muddebihal, MDS, Krishna A. Rao, MDS and Khaled Elrahawy, PhD
Oral Pathology, Preventive Dentistry Department,
College of Dentistry, Jouf University, Aljouf, Saudi Arabia

Oral biology is a specialized area of dentistry that deals and establishes sound basic knowledge of oral and paraoral tissues and structures. It introduces basic concepts of growth and development, maturational and aging processes of tissues, systems within craniofacial complex and deviation and variation from the normal growth and development and prepares a student for preclinical and clinical stages. It also helps in understanding the role of genetics, hormones and nutrition in growth and development. Having a thorough knowledge of oral biology helps the students in understanding the pathogenesis and underlying pathosis and accordingly plan an appropriate treatment procedure including prevention of the further progress of the disease process.

This chapter has been prepared keeping this in mind and would definitely serve as a valuable guide to students of various disciplines. It provides an overview of various aspects of oral biology in the form of scenario-based questions focusing essentially on learning and understanding concepts rather than illogical way of memorization. Though oral biology is a preclinical subject, in this chapter, we have made a sincere effort to provide the students with careful, methodically prepared, scenario-based questions as far as possible.

1. The Mandibular processes merge or fuse with each other at midline by end of
   - **A. 4th week intrauterine life**
   - B. 8th week intrauterine life
   - C. 2nd week intrauterine life
   - D. 6th week intrauterine life

2. Intermaxillary segment is formed by fusion of
   - A. Two Maxillary processes
   - B. Two Mandibular processes
   - C. Two Lateral nasal processes
   - **D. Two Medial nasal processes**

3. Teeth begin to develop at
   - A. 2nd week intrauterine life
   - B. 4th week intrauterine life
   - **C. 6th week intrauterine life**
   - D. 8th week intrauterine life

4. Tooth crown assumes its final shape in the
   - A. Bud stage
   - B. Cap stage
   - **C. Early bell stage**
   - D. Advanced bell stage

5. True denticles contain
    A. Dentinal tubules
    B. Dentinal fluid
    C. Dentinal nerves
    D. Dentinal vessels

6. Around the teeth which have lost their antagonists
    A. Cancellous bone around the alveolus is reduced and the trabeculae become less numerous and very thin
    B. Cancellous bone around the alveolus is increased and the trabeculae become more numerous and very thick
    C. Remains the same without any changes
    D. All of the above are false

7. Pink spots seen in the crown of a mandibular molar are diagnostic of:
    A. Irreversible pulpitis
    B. Calcific metamorphosis
    C. Internal root resorption
    D. Pulp stones

8. Over the cusps of teeth the rods appear twisted around each other in a seemingly complex arrangement known as
    A. Hunter-Schreger Bands
    B. Gnarled Enamel
    C. Enamel tufts
    D. Enamel lamellae

9. Nerve supply to oral mucous membrane includes all the following nerves *except*
    A. Trochlear
    B. Trigeminal
    C. Glossopharyngeal
    D. Vagus

10. Birbeck granules are seen in
    - A. Melanocytes
    - **B. Langerhans cells**
    - C. Merkel cells
    - D. Inflammatory cells

11. Epithelial attachment includes
    - A. Basal lamina & Desmosomes
    - B. Desmosomes & gap junctions
    - C. Desmosomes & hemidesmosomes
    - **D. Basal lamina & hemidesmosomes**

12. In the fourth stage of passive eruption
    - A. Anatomical crown is larger than clinical crown
    - **B. Clinical crown is larger than anatomical crown**
    - C. Clinical crown & anatomical crown are equal in length
    - D. Clinical is not related to passive eruption

13. Clinical crown is equal to anatomical crown in which stage of passive eruption?
    - A. First stage
    - B. Second stage
    - **C. Third stage**
    - D. Fourth stage

14. The successional lamina when developed in the fifth month in utero gives rise to which tooth?
    - A. Deciduous central incisor
    - B. Permanent lateral incisor
    - C. Deciduous lateral incisor
    - **D. Permanent central incisor**

15. When a longitudinal ground section of tooth is observed under oblique reflected light, a change in direction of rods is noted in the form of dark and light bands. Identify the term used to describe such alternate bands?
    A. Incremental lines of Retzius
    B. Incremental lines of Von Ebner
    C. Hunter-Schreger bands
    D. Enamel lamellae

16. Saliva contains which of the following immunoglobins?
    A. Ig A
    B. Ig G
    C. Ig E
    D. Ig F

17. Identify which of the following functions as a shock absorber?
    A. Maxilla
    B. Mandible
    C. TMJ
    D. Salivary gland

18. During the first week of prenatal developmental 16-celled structure called as morula resembles a,
    A. Raspberry
    B. Mulberry
    C. Strawberry
    D. Grapes

19. Which is the most critical or dangerous period in a pregnant woman?
    A. Germinal period.
    B. Organogenetic period
    C. Fetal period
    D. Implantation period

20. Which cells are involved in formation of dentin?
    A. Ameloblasts
    B. Odontoblasts
    C. Dentinoblasts
    D. Cementoblasts

21. An infant is brought to a dental clinic due to problems in suckling. On intraoral examination, the tongue was bifid. The probable cause for the development of such pathology is due to failure of fusion of
    A. The two lateral lingual swellings
    B. The lingual swellings and tuberculum impar
    C. Hypobranchial eminence and tuberculum impar
    D. Hypobranchial eminence and lingual swellings

22. During which of the following stages of the life cycle of ameloblasts, dentin formation begins?
    A. Morphogenic stage
    B. Organizing stage
    C. Formative stage
    D. Maturative stage

23. Odontoblasts develop from
    A. Inner enamel epithelium
    B. Dental sac
    C. Outer enamel epithelium
    D. Dental papilla

24. Neonatal line is seen in
    A. Permanent teeth only
    B. Deciduous teeth only
    C. All permanent teeth and deciduous first molars
    D. All deciduous teeth and permanent first molars

25. In the absence of development of teeth (Anodontia), which of the following statements is true?
    A. Only development of the basal bone gets affected
    B. Only development of the alveolar bone gets affected
    C. Development of both basal bone and alveolar bone gets affected
    D. Neither is affected as their growth is independent of tooth development

26. On a radiograph, the alveolar bone proper is described as
    A. Lamina lucida
    B. Lamina limitans
    C. Lamina propria
    D. Lamina dura

27. A patient presents to the dental clinic with a complaint of absence of multiple teeth. This phenomenon is likely to occur due to a disturbance in which of the following physiological stages of tooth development?
    A. Proliferation
    B. Initiation
    C. Histodifferentiation
    D. Morphodifferentiation

28. Which of the following conditions shows multiple supernumerary teeth?
    A. Dentin dysplasia
    B. Regional odontodysplasia
    C. Epithelial dysplasia
    D. Cleidocranial dysplasia

29. Which of the following is the most common missing tooth?
    - A. Maxillary first premolar.
    - **B. Maxillary permanent lateral incisor**
    - C. Maxillary permanent central incisor
    - D. Maxillary second premolar

30. Which of the following is not a feature of Hutchinson's triad?
    - **A. Intestinal keratosis**
    - B. VIII nerve deafness
    - C. Enamel hypoplasia of permanent incisors and molars
    - D. Interstitial keratitis

31. A 23-year-old patient complained of multiple loose teeth. On clinical examination, nothing abnormal was detected with well-maintained oral hygiene. However, on radiographic examination, the periodontal status was healthy and all teeth had conical and abnormally short roots. The diagnosis is likely to be
    - A. Dentin hypocalcification
    - B. Dentinogenesis imperfecta
    - C. Hypophosphatasia
    - **D. Dentin dysplasia**

32. Which of the following is predominantly a serous salivary gland?
    - **A. Parotid gland in a new born infant**
    - B. Parotid gland in an adult
    - C. Von Ebner's gland
    - D. Glossopalatine glands

33. Which of the following cells of the salivary glands is responsible for the controlled flow of the saliva?
    - A. Serous cells
    - B. Mucus cells
    - **C. Myoepithelial cells**
    - D. Ductal cells

34. Which of the following cells do not contribute in the formation of saliva?
    A. Cells of the excretory duct
    B. Cells of the striated duct
    C. Mucous cells
    D. Serous cells

35. Mucoperiosteum may be seen in
    A. Gingival mucosa
    B. Alveolar mucosa
    C. Buccal mucosa
    D. Labial mucosa

36. Which of the following may not be a function of oral mucosa in human beings?
    A. Protection
    B. Sensation
    C. Secretion
    D. Thermoregulation

37. Which of the following layers of the oral epithelium is important for maintaining the structural integrity of the oral epithelium?
    A. Stratum corneum
    B. Stratum basale
    C. Stratum spinosum
    D. Stratum granulosum

38. Which of the following cells play a role in defense of oral mucosa by phagocytosis?
    A. Merkel cells
    B. Melanocytes
    C. Langerhans cells
    D. Lymphocytes

39. Which component of the basal lamina is affected in bullous pemphigoid?
    - **A. Lamina lucida**
    - B. Lamina propria
    - C. Lamina densa
    - D. Sublamina densa

40. Synovial fluid in the joint space of TMJ is maintained by
    - A. Intermediate cells
    - B. Vascular intima
    - C. Type A cells
    - **D. Type B cells**

41. Which of the following nerve endings help in proprioception in TMJ?
    - A. Ruffini's corpuscles
    - B. Pacinian corpuscles
    - C. **Golgi tendon**
    - D. Noci receptors

42. Lower joint cavity of TMJ assists in
    - A. Forward movement of the mandible
    - B. Backward movement of the mandible
    - **C. Lowering and elevating the mandible**
    - D. Lateral movement of the mandible

43. The apex of the maxillary sinus is towards the
    - A. Lateral wall of the nasal cavity
    - **B. Zygomatic process**
    - C. Orbital floor
    - D. Alveolar process

44. In a haematoxylin and eosin stained histological section of salivary gland, lightly stained pyramidal cells with flat nuclei arranged in tubular pattern are noted. These cells could be
    A. Ductal cells
    B. Myoepithelial cells
    C. Serous cells
    D. Mucous cells

45. All of the following cells produce collagen fibres *except*
    A. Ameloblasts
    B. Odontoblasts
    C. Chondroblasts
    D. Osteoblasts

46. When an oral surgeon extracts a mandibular first molar, all of the principal fibers of the periodontal ligament are torn from their attachment to alveolar bone *except* for the
    A. Transeptal fibers
    B. Oblique fibers
    C. Interradicular fibers
    D. Dentoperiosteal fibers

47. Which type of dentin is produced throughout the life of an individual?
    A. Intratubular dentin
    B. Interglobular dentin
    C. Tertiary dentin
    D. Mantle dentin

48. When a tooth first erupts into the oral cavity, the attachment epithelial cuff is composed of epithelium derived from
    A. Dental lamina
    B. Epithelial rests of Malassez
    C. Reduced dental epithelium
    D. Hertwig's Epithelial root sheath

49. 13-year-old girl presents to a general dentist with a chipped upper central incisor with a history of trauma the previous day. She complains of pain in tooth while drinking cold water. On clinical examination, the tooth exhibited fractured Enamel along with the underlying intact Dentin. Depending on this, which part or content of the dentinal tubule is responsible for pain felt by the patient?
    A. Dentinal Fluid
    B. Odontoblastic process
    C. Nerve endings
    D. Odontoblasts receptors

50. The histology of enamel can be best studied by which of the following methods:
    A. Decalcified H & E stain
    B. Ground section
    C. PAS stain
    D. Exfoliative cytology

51. Identify which is not a part of or arise from the dental organ
    A. Reduced enamel epithelium
    B. Dental sac
    C. Cervical loop
    D. Epithelial root sheath

52. If the dentist drills deep into a tooth and exposes the pulp chamber, and reassures the patient by placing calcium hydroxide cement, then which of the following cells of the pulp are more responsible for healing and repair in this area?
    A. Mast cell
    B. Odontoblast
    C. Fibroblast
    D. Undifferentiated cell

53. Mandible ossification starts in which of the following regions?
    - A. Symphysis menti
    - B. Condyle
    - **C. Mental foramen**
    - D. Coronoid

54. The presence of Tomes' processes is associated with the
    - A. Formation of peritubular dentin
    - B. Morphogenic function of dental organ
    - C. **Secretory function of dental organ**
    - D. Hypomineralized root dentin

55. Specific gravity of enamel is
    - A. 2.2
    - **B. 2.8**
    - C. 2.9
    - D. 2.7

56. Tooth calcification is disturbed if a child is ill for a long period of time. Which of the following stages of tooth development gets affected?
    - A. Bud stage
    - B. Cap stage
    - C. Early bell stage
    - **D. Late bell stage**

57. Which of the following structures was considered to be an optical phenomenon?
    - A. Line of Retzius
    - B. Spindle
    - C. Tufts
    - **D. Hunter-Schreger bands**

58. All of the following tissues are mesenchymal in origin *except*
    - A. Dentin
    - B. Pulp
    - C. Cementum
    - **D. Enamel**

59. All of the following factors may contribute to the normal color of the oral mucosa *except*
    - A. Degree of keratinization
    - B. Thickness of the epithelium
    - **C. Attachment of the epithelium**
    - D. Vascularity of the tissue

60. Lamina limitans is
    - **A. The organic membrane present on the inner wall of the dentinal tubule**
    - B. Alveolar bone proper
    - C. Supporting alveolar bone
    - D. Supporting connective tissue of the oral mucous membrane

61. Thin, dark, leaf-like structures seen in enamel in longitudinal sections are
    - A. Enamel spindles
    - **B. Enamel lamellae**
    - C. Enamel tufts
    - D. Enamel niche

62. Which of the following structures related to dentin may extend into enamel?
    - A. Intratubular nerves
    - B. Intertubular nerves
    - **C. Odontoblastic process**
    - D. Interglobular dentin

63. During active dentinogenesis, the pulpward movement of the odontoblasts is achieved due to the presence of
    A. Odontoblastic layer
    B. Cell-free zone
    C. Cell-rich zone
    D. Parietal layer

64. Which of the following tissues undergoes resorption under physiological condition?
    A. Cementum
    B. Enamel
    C. Dentin
    D. Bone

65. Ankylosis of tooth may result from resorption of
    A. Periodontal ligament
    B. Alveolar bone
    C. Cementum
    D. Dentin

66. Of the principal group of fibers of the periodontal ligament, the most numerous are
    A. Alveolar crest group
    B. Oblique group
    C. Horizontal group
    D. Apical group

67. Reversal of nutritional/blood supply is seen in
    A. Morphogenic stage
    B. Formative stage
    C. Maturative stage
    D. Organizing Stage

68. Which of the following is keratinized?
    A. Gingival Col
    B. Sulcular epithelium
    C. Attached gingiva
    D. Junctional epithelium

69. The most critical stage of life cycle of ameloblasts is
    A. Organizing stage
    B. Protective stage
    C. Desmolytic stage
    D. Formative stage

70. Which of the following lingual papilla is heavily keratinized?
    A. Fungiform papilla
    B. Filiform papilla
    C. Circumvallate papilla
    D. Foliate papilla

71. The special sensory nerve supply to the circumvallate papilla is through
    A. Lingual nerve
    B. Chorda tympani
    C. Glossopharyngeal nerve
    D. Hypoglossal nerve

72. Odland body
    A. Is a special sensory cell present in the oral epithelium
    B. Helps in thermoregulation
    C. Contributes in oral secretion
    D. Protects the deeper tissues by forming a physical barrier

73. The mucous membrane is thinnest in
    A. Ventral surface of tongue and floor of the mouth
    B. Lips and cheeks

C. Gingiva and alveolar mucosa
D. Hard and soft palates

74. A zone that is exclusively seen only in human beings and not in other mammals is
A. Buccal mucosa
B. Labial mucosa
C. Vermilion border
D. Palatal mucosa

75. Gubernacular canal is seen during
A. Pre-eruptive phase
B. Eruptive phase
C. Post eruptive phase
D. Post-functional phase

REFERENCES

Avery, James K. *Essentials of Oral Histology and amp.; Embryology,* 3rd Edition.
Berkovitz, B.K.B. *Oral Anatomy, Histology and amp.; Embryology,* 4th Edition.
Chiego, Daniel J. *Essentials of Oral Histology and amp.; Embryology: A Clinical Approach*, 4th Edition.
Kumar, G.S. *Orban's Oral Histology and amp.; Embryology,* 14th Edition.
Nanci, Antonio. *Ten Cate's Oral Histology*, 8th Edition.

In: Scenario Based MCQ in Dentistry ISBN: 978-1-53617-298-0
Editors: M. Khursheed Alam et al. © 2020 Nova Science Publishers, Inc.

Chapter 13

SCENARIO BASED MCQS IN ORAL PATHOLOGY

Manay Srinivas Munisekhar, MDS, Farahnaz Muddebihal, MDS, Krishna A. Rao, MDS and Khaled Elrahawy, PhD

Oral Pathology, Preventive Dentistry Department,
College of Dentistry, Jouf University, Aljouf, Saudi Arabia

Oral and Maxillofacial Pathology is a specialized branch of dentistry that is concerned with the diagnosis of the diseases of the oral cavity, jaws, and the associated structures such as the temporomandibular joint, salivary glands, oral and perioral musculature, and skin. It also deals with the causes and the effects of the diseases in the maxillofacial complex. It forms the basis for clinical dentistry. Rightfully, it is reflected in the curriculum of the dentistry program where it is sandwiched between the basic sciences and clinical branches of dentistry.

It is only after a thorough understanding of oral and maxillofacial pathology, that a clinical practitioner can diagnose a disease more accurately and institute an appropriate treatment. Without an apt knowledge of oral pathology, one cannot become a successful clinician.

Consistent with this concept, most of the clinical situations that we routinely encounter have been carefully structured as scenario-based questions that activate the cognitive skills of the reader to correctly answer the questions.

In this chapter, the questions are intentionally not sequenced topic-wise so as to challenge the reader. Moreover, the options are prepared meticulously and are require nearly the same critical thinking and high-minded judgement. A sincere effort was made not to copy, repeat, or design scenarios.

1. A tanned, 66-year old man presents with an ulcerated lesion on the nose, with a rolled edge. The incisional biopsy revealed nests & cords of cuboidal cells with palisaded appearance of the peripheral neoplastic cells. The most likely diagnosis is
    A. Aphthous ulcer
    B. Basal cell carcinoma
    C. Tuberculous ulcer
    D. Bowen's disease

2. A 60-year old man complains of a bleeding ulcer on the upper region of the left cheek. It as an everted edge and there are some palpable cervical lymph nodes. On examination, the histopathological features showed invasion of overlying epithelium into subjacent structures in the form of small nests of hyperchromatic cells exhibiting few mitotic figures, cellular & nuclear pleomorphism along with islands of keratinization. The above mentioned features are suggestive of
    A. Verrucous carcinoma
    B. Basal cell carcinoma
    C. Squamous cell carcinoma
    D. Malignant melanoma

3. A 33-year old man presents with the swelling on the upper arm which has been growing slowly for a number of years. Examination reveals a small, compressible, non-tender, lobulated mass and histopathology shows adipocytes enclosed within areolar tissue surrounded by a fibrous capsule. The most likely lesion to reveal these features is
    A. Lipoma
    B. Fibroma
    C. Neurofibroma
    D. Osteoma

4. A 30-year-old female presents with slowly growing, submucosal mass on the dorsal surface of the tongue that is painless and freely movable. The histopathological examination shows a highly cellular stroma made of spindle cells arranged in two different patterns along with Verocay bodies. The immunohistochemical examination shows positivity for S 100 protein. The most probable lesion would be
    A. Spindle cell carcinoma
    B. Verruca vulgaris
    C. Schwannoma
    D. Leiomyoma

5. A 29-year-old man presents with multiple fusiform shaped lumps on the forearm with café-au-lait pigmentations on the skin. Each swelling firm rubbery in consistency and causes tingling in the hand upon pressure. The biopsy examination shows spindle shaped cells with fusiform or wavy nuclei scattered in delicate, myxoid connective tissue stroma containing numerous mast cells. All the features are suggestive of
    A. Multiple Myeloma
    B. Multiple Neurilemmoma
    C. Multiple Lipoma
    D. Multiple Neurofibroma

6. A 45-year-old male with the habit of tobacco chewing since 20 years presents with an unilateral white patch in the buccal vestibule that cannot be scrapped. The incisional biopsy reveals a dysplastic, hyperorthokeratotic, hyperplastic epithelium with an inflamed CT stroma. The most likely lesion to cause this would be
   A. Leukoplakia
   B. Squamous acanthoma
   C. Frictional keratosis
   D. Lichen planus

7. A 50-year-old female presents with bilateral white patches on the buccal mucosa showing Wickham's striae radiating from the patches. The histopathology shows hyperkeratosis, saw-tooth shaped rete ridges of the epithelium with basal cell degeneration. The epithelium-CT interface shows dense chronic inflammatory cell infiltrate. The above mentioned features indicate the lesion to be
   A. White spongy nevus
   B. Lichen planus
   C. Leukoplakia
   D. Frictional keratosis

8. An elderly individual about 65 years of age with severe diabetes and immunocompromised condition presents with a diffuse white patch below the denture. The white patch can be easily scrapped off leaving a red erythematous area. The histopathology showed slender, eosinophilic, hyphae-like structures which is PAS positive. The underlying CT shows severe chronic inflammatory cell infiltrate. It is most likely to be
   A. Lichen planus
   B. Candidiasis
   C. Leukoplakia
   D. White spongy nevus

9. A 40-year-old male presents with an asymptomatic, firm, submucosal swelling in the palatal region showing a wide spectrum of histopathological features. The lesion has a poorly defined capsule with varying proportion of ductal and myoepithelial cells scattered in a background of myxoid, hyalinized CT stroma. The plasmacytoid cells or spindle cells in the lesion show immunoprofile co-expresson of cytokeratin markers, vimentin, calponin, alpha smooth muscle actin and muscle-specific actin. The lesion exhibiting the above features can be diagnosed as
   A. Oncocytoma
   B. Monomorphic adenoma
   C. Ductal papilloma
   D. Pleomorphic adenoma

10. A 62-year-old male with a history of smoking since 40 years complains of a painless, firm swelling in the right cheek region. On examination, the swelling was around 3x4 cm in size with well-defined borders. Microscopic features revealed cyst formation with papillary projections into cystic spaces exhibiting lymphoid matrix with germinal centers. The cysts were lined by papillary proliferations of bi-layered oncocytic epithelium. The most likely diagnosis of the lesion would be
    A. Warthin's tumour
    B. Pleomorphic adenoma
    C. Squamous papilloma
    D. Basal cell adenoma

11. A 25-year-old patient presented with a swelling in the lower right posterior part of the jaw. Radiological examination revealed multilocular radiolucency with scalloped border causing displacement of 46 and 47. FNAC revealed a thin straw colored fluid. Microscopic features revealed a cystic space line by uniformly thick parakeratinzed epithelium exhibiting picket fence appearance of basal cell layer. The surface of the epithelium showed corrugations and the underlying

connective tissue was mildly inflamed. Along with the clinical correlation the histopathological features are suggestive of

A. Keratocysticodontogenic tumor
B. Calcifying epithelial odontogenic cyst
C. Sialo-odontogenic cyst
D. Adamantinoma

12. A 33-year-old patient exhibited an asymptomatic swelling in the mandibular left posterior region with facial deformity. On palpation there was crepitus or egg shell cracking of the involved cortical plates. Radiological features demonstrated a multiloculated soap bubble appearance along with resorption of roots of involved teeth. Histopathological features showed follicular type of arrangement exhibiting peripheral columnar cells with palisaded arrangement along with loosely arranged stellate shaped cells in the center. The surrounding CT stroma exhibited moderate to densely packed collagen fiber bundles. These features suggest that the lesion could be

A. Squamous odontogenic tumor
B. Calcifying epithelial odontogenic tumor
C. Adenomatoid odontogenic Tumor
D. Ameloblastoma

13. A 25-year-old female patient presented with an asymptomatic, vividly erythematous discrete macules, papules with occasional vesicles and bullae distributed in symmetrical pattern over the upper and lower limbs. A characteristic iris-like lesions with varying shades of erythema could be noticed. The histopathological features showed intracellular edema of spinous cell layer of the epithelium with subepidermal vesicle. There was also dilatation of superficial capillaries and lymphatic vessels in the uppermost part of CT with varying degree of inflammatory cell infiltration. The histopathological features along with clinical correlation is suggestive of

A. Psoriasis
B. Pemphigus vulgaris

C. Erythema multiforme
D. Epidermolysisbullosa

14. A condition where bull-like teeth are present is referred to as,
    A. Macrodontia
    B. Taurodontism
    C. Talons cusp
    D. Gemination

15. A 25-year-old male patient visited a dental clinic with a complaint of sharp pain while chewing food. Clinical examination revealed presence of generalized attrition. A radiograph investigation suggested of no obvious caries or any other pathology. Identify the lesion?
    A. Avulsion.
    B. Dilaceration
    C. Cracked tooth syndrome
    D. Concrescence

16. A 25-year-old female complains of painless swelling on lower lip with a history of accidental lip biting. On examination it was a dome shaped swelling with a size of about 1mm in diameter. The pathology report suggested of pools of mucus and granulation tissue with lobules of minor salivary gland. The most likely diagnosis could be
    A. Mucocele
    B. Ranula
    C. Pleomorphic adenoma
    D. Traumatic bone cyst

17. Lichen Planus is associated with which of the following syndromes?
    A. Grinspan syndrome
    B. Kelly-Patterson Syndrome
    C. Down's syndrome
    D. Peutz-Jeghers syndrome

18. A 35-year-old male reported to a dental clinic with slow growing swelling on tongue. The pathology report suggested of an encapsulated tumor containing Antoni A and Antoni B types of cells. Identify what is the lesion?
    A. Squamous papilloma
    B. Schwannoma
    C. Neurofibroma
    D. Leiomyoma

19. A 4-year child was brought to the dental clinic with a complaint of multiple decayed teeth. On examination, multiple carious teeth were noted involving all four quadrants of the jaws sparing the lower anteriors. The most likely diagnosis is
    A. Rampant caries
    B. Acute caries
    C. Primary caries
    D. Nursing bottle caries

20. A 25-year-old male patient presented with severe continuous pain in the lower left back tooth. On intraoral examination, 36 was found to be associated with a large restoration with defective margins. The condition is more likely to be
    A. Acute closed pulpitis
    B. Acute open pulpitis
    C. Chronic closed pulpitis
    D. Chronic open pulpitis

21. An 8-year-old male patient was brought to a dental clinic with a complaint of carious tooth and a mass within the carious tooth. On clinical examination, 46 was involved with a large carious defect and with a pinkish-red globular tissue protruding from the pulp chamber. The diagnosis is
    A. Chronic ulcerative pulpitis
    B. Chronic hyperplastic pulpitis

C. Focal pulpal hyperemia
D. Chronic closed pulpitis

22. A male patient aged 25 years presented with mild tooth pain and a bony hard welling of the jaw. The tooth associated (36) was non-vital and on radiographic examination, intraoral periapical radiograph showed a radio-opaque mass associated with 36 and the occlusal radiograph showed revealed a focal overgrowth of bone on the outer surface of the cortex. The condition is most likely to be
   A. Acute osteomyelitis
   B. Condensing osteitis
   C. Garre's osteomyelitis
   D. Chronic diffuse sclerosing osteomyelitis

23. A 40-year-old patient presented to the dental clinic with fever, diffuse painful swelling of the soft tissues of the face, the overlying skin was inflamed and red, and regional lymphadenitis. On examination, there was trismus and 46 was associated with deep dental caries and was non vital. The likely diagnosis is
   A. Cellulitis
   B. Acute closed pulpitis
   C. Acute apical periodontitis
   D. Acute suppurative osteomyelitis

24. A 25-year-old female patient visited a dental clinic with severe trismus and radiating pain. On clinical examination, pericoronitis was noted without any evidence of clinical facial swelling. This may be an indicative that the infection has spread to
   A. Submasseteric space
   B. Pterygomandibular space
   C. Retropharyngeal space
   D. Infratemporal space

25. A one and half year-old infant was brought to the dental clinic due to absence of teeth in the oral cavity. On general examination, the infant was diminutive or small for her age, the hair was sparse and silky, skin was dry, wrinkled and atrophic. On radiographic examination, all teeth related were present within the jaws. The diagnosis of the condition is
    A. Ectodermal dysplasia
    B. Hypopituitarism
    C. Hyperpituitarism
    D. Hyperthyroidism

26. A 40-year-old patient presented to the dental clinic with a brown flushy mass intra-orally for the last 1 month. Laboratory investigations revealed increased calcium and alkaline phosphatase levels in the serum. Whole body scans revealed renal stones and gall bladder stones. Radiographs revealed multiple osteolytic lesions in the skull and jaws. Histopathology showed multinucleated giant cells scattered within a delicate connective tissue. The likely diagnosis is
    A. Central giant cell granuloma
    B. Peripheral giant cell granuloma
    C. Hyperparathyroidism
    D. Giant cell tumor

27. A patient complained of white patch and burning sensation in the right cheek. On examination, reticular white radiating lesion was noted and 47 and 48 were decayed and filled with amalgam. The possible diagnosis is
    A. Leukoplakia
    B. Lichen planus
    C. Lichenoid reaction
    D. Leukedema

28. A 6-year-old child was brought to a dentist with prolonged and massive bleeding in the oral cavity for the last 24 hrs. History revealed that the child has a tendency to bleed easily and that the present

episode followed normal exfoliation of lower anterior tooth. On investigation, his bleeding time was normal and clotting time was prolonged. The diagnosis is

A. von Willebrand's disease
B. Factor XII deficiency
C. Factor X deficiency
D. **Hemophilia**

29. The difference between malignant ameloblastoma and ameloblastic carcinoma is that in malignant ameloblastoma, the metastatic lesion:

A. Bears no resemblance to primary tumor
B. Shows no significant histologic difference from the primary tumor
C. Shows histologic difference from primary tumor
D. None of the above. Both are synonymous

30. Examination of 3-year-old boy reveals a fracture of his right leg, blue sclera and peculiarly shaped head. Opalescent dentin is found in majority of his primary teeth. Most probable diagnosis is:

A. Osteopetrosis
B. Osteitis deformans
C. Osteogenesis imperfecta
D. Infantile cortical hyperostosis

31. A young girl presents with an expansile mass in left maxillary region which was seen as radiopaque, poorly demarcated, finely trabeculated mass on radiographic examination. Histopathologic examination shows randomly distributed spicules of osteoid scattered throughout a young connective tissue stroma. Most suggestive diagnosis of the lesion is:

A. Fibrous dysplasia
B. Paget's disease
C. Osteosarcoma
D. Osteopetrosis

32. Which of the following histological types of ameloblastoma shows marked tendency for recurrence and shows aggressive behavior?
    A. Follicular
    B. Plexiform
    C. Acanthomatous
    D. Granular cell

33. Which of the following types of nevi occur most frequently in the oral cavity?
    A. Intradermal nevus
    B. Junctional nevus
    C. Compound nevus
    D. Blue nevus

34. Most characteristic histopathologic feature of Keratoacanthoma is:
    A. Elevation of normal epithelium toward the central portion of the lesion with an abrupt change in normal epithelium as hyperplastic acanthotic epithelium is reached
    B. Hyperplastic squamous epithelium growing into underlying connective tissue
    C. Occasional dysplastic feature
    D. Epithelium appears to be invading into connective tissue at deep leading margin of the tumor

35. Elevated serum alkaline phosphatase levels may be seen in:
    A. Paget's disease
    B. Caffey's disease
    C. Severe polyostotic fibrous dysplasia
    D. Any of the above

36. Clinically and histologically keratoacanthoma may closely resemble:
    A. Basal cell carcinoma
    B. Squamous cell carcinoma

C. Malignant melanoma
D. Leukoplakia

37. Nevus cells are believed to be derived from:
    A. Yolk sac
    B. Ectoderm
    C. Neural crest
    D. Mesoderm

38. The site most commonly affected by basal cell carcinoma is:
    A. Buccal mucosa
    B. Skin of palm and exposed surface of arms
    C. Skin of upper back area
    D. Skin of middle third of face

39. Virus which may cause Burkitt's lymphoma is:
    A. Herpes simplex virus type II
    B. Cytomegalovirus
    C. Epstien-Barr virus
    D. Varicella Zoster virus

40. The sites most commonly affected by malignant melanoma are:
    A. Buccal mucosa and palate
    B. Mandibular and maxillary gingivae
    C. Palate and maxillary gingiva
    D. Palate and tongue

41. The reasons for red appearance of lesion of erythroplakia are:
    A. Connective tissue pegs extending very high into the epithelium and epithelium being thin over tips of CT papillae
    B. Absence of significance amount of ortho or parakeratinised layer
    C. Dilation of capillaries in connective tissue pegs
    D. All of the above

42. A definitive diagnosis of oral hairy leukoplakia requires the
    A. Demonstration of Coxsackie A group virus
    B. Demonstration of Epstein-Barr virus-DNA
    C. Absence of koilocytes in the spinous cell layer
    D. Presence of Oral Herpes virus

43. Which of the following is uncommon in oral mucosa?
    A. Squamous papilloma
    B. Fibroma
    C. Verruca vulgaris
    D. Hemangioma

44. Histologic examination of lesion of oral submucous fibrosis shows all of the following *except*
    A. Epithelial atrophy and loss of retepegs
    B. Epithelial atypia
    C. Hyalinization of connective tissue
    D. Epithelial hypertrophy

45. All of the following statements concerning osteosarcoma are true *except*
    A. It is a malignant bone tumor composed of anaplastic cells derived from mesenchyme
    B. Its peak incidence is after epiphyseal fusion, particularly the year between 50 and 60
    C. This tumor seems to arise in the long bones which show the greatest longitudinal growth
    D. Joint involvement is rare

46. A 25-year-old patient presents with smooth enlargement of body of mandible in right molar region which is present for last 1 ½ years and in slowly and steadily increasing in size. The most probable diagnosis is:
    A. Adenomatoidodontogenic tumor

B. Mucocele

C. Ameloblastoma

D. Peripheral giant cell granuloma

47. A 20-year-old patient came to the dental clinic with a swelling in relation to 11 and 21. Clinically 11 and 21 were discolored and the history revealed that there was trauma 10 years ago while playing football. The likely diagnosis is

A. Odontogenic keratocyst

B. Dentigerous cyst

C. Radicular cyst

D. Nasopalatine cyst

48. A 6-month old infant is brought to the clinic due to defective upper lip. On examination, the patient had median cleft lip. This occurs due to failure of fusion of

A. Two medial nasal processes

B. Medial and lateral nasal processes

C. Medial nasal process and maxillary process

D. Lateral nasal process and maxillary process

49. A 16 year old patient visits a dental clinician with a complaint of swelling and pain just prior to, during and after food intake in the retromandibular region on the left side. On intraoral examination, 37 showed a deep carious lesion and an unerupted 38. The diagnosis is more likely to be a

A. Radicular cyst

B. Sialolithiasis

C. Impacted third molar

D. Acute pulpitis

50. A 6 year old child presented with generalized defects of all teeth present in the oral cavity with defective vertical grooves on the surface of the tooth. The possible diagnosis is
    A. **Amelogenesis imperfecta**
    B. Environmental enamel hypoplasia
    C. Dentinogenesis imperfecta
    D. Regional odontodysplasia

51. A 20 year old female patient presented with maxillary anterior swelling with a retained deciduous maxillary canine on the right side. On radiographic examination, a pericoronal radiolucency surrounding the crown of an impacted permanent canine was seen. The most likely diagnosis
    A. Pindborg's tumor
    B. Ameloblastoma
    C. Periapicalcemental dysplasia
    D. **Adenomatoid odontogenic tumor**

52. A patient complained of pus discharge from the opening of the Stensen's duct on the right side. The patient is diagnosed with
    A. Viral sialadenitis
    B. **Bacterial sialadenitis**
    C. Allergic sialadenitis
    D. Sarcoid sialadenitis

53. A patient presented with facial paralysis and parotid swelling on the right side. The diagnosis is more likely to be
    A. Pleomorphic adenoma
    B. Mucoepidermoid carcinoma
    C. **Adenoid cystic carcinoma**
    D. Warthin's tumor

54. Which of the following is the most common odontogenic tumor?
    A. Ameloblastoma
    B. Adenomatoid odontogenic tumor
    C. Pindborg's tumor
    D. Odontoma

55. A female patient complained of burning mouth and on examination, a bilateral, non-scrapable white lesion was noticed on the buccal mucosa. The history also revealed that she did not have any deleterious habits and that she was medically fit. The most likely diagnosis could be
    A. Lichen planus
    B. Leukoplakia
    C. Frictional keratosis
    D. Lichenoid reaction

56. An adult male patient presented with vesicles on the skin that were characteristically unilateral and did not cross the midline. It is most likely to be
    A. Herpes simplex
    B. Herpes zoster
    C. Chicken pox
    D. Small pox

57. A patient presented with continuous pain and swelling in the left lower back tooth. On clinical examination, 36 was decayed with pulpal involvement and it was tender on vertical percussion. The diagnosis is
    A. Acute irreversible pulpitis
    B. Reversible pulpitis
    C. Acute apical periodontitis
    D. Chronic reversible pulpitis

58. An elderly patient complains of the need to change his dentures and hats frequently due to progressive enlargement of the bones of the cranium and facial skeleton. The best possible diagnosis could be
    A. Fibrous dysplasia of bone
    B. Cleidocranial dysplasia
    C. Infantile cortical hyperostosis
    D. Paget's disease

59. An 8-year-old child presents with gingivitis, gingival enlargement, gingival hemorrhage and necrotic gingival ulcers. The child may be suffering from
    A. Acute necrotizing ulcerative gingivitis
    B. Inflammatory gingival enlargement
    C. Leukemia
    D. Vitamin C deficiency

60. A child patient is being reported to the dentist for deformities in teeth. On clinical examination, the patient had very little hair, dry skin, many missing teeth for his age and malformed teeth. On careful history, the attendant of the patient revealed repeated bouts of unexplained fever and absence of sweating on physical activity. The child is likely to be suffering from
    A. Anodontia
    B. Regional odontodysplasia
    C. Ectodermal dysplasia
    D. Vitamin D deficiency

61. A patient presented with extensive skin involvement with vesicles and bullae to the clinic. On clinical examination, there was loss of skin on digital pressure. Immunofluorescence revealed a fish-net pattern of fluorescence. The likely diagnosis is
    A. Benign mucous membrane pemphigoid
    B. Bullous pemphigoid

C. Cicatricial pemphigoid

D. Pemphigus

62. A female patient complains of frequent bleeding and superficial ulcerations of the oral mucosa. On general examination, she had erythematous patches on the face which was characteristically butterfly shaped distribution. The likely diagnosis is

A. Vitamin K deficiency

B. Vitamin C deficiency

C. Neutropenia

D. Systemic lupus erythematosus

63. Which one of the following was thought to be a developmental anomaly earlier but is now suggested to be associated with candida albicans? Clinically, it is seen on the midline of the dorsal surface of the tongue and devoid of filiform papillae:

A. Median rhomboid glossitis

B. Geographic tongue

C. Fissured tongue

D. Lingual thyroid

64. The exotoses that are found on the lingual aspect of the mandible in the area of the premolars bilaterally are referred to as:

A. Mandibular tori

B. Lingual mandibular bone concavity

C. Genial tubercles

D. Mandibular fossa

65. A small fluid-filled, circumscribed lesion usually less than 1cm in diameter that is elevated and protrudes above the surface of normal surrounding tissue is called a:

A. Bulla

B. Macule

C. **Vesicle**

D. Papule

66. Which one the following is characterized by abnormal increase in the circulating RBC?
    A. Leukopenia
    B. Polydipsia
    C. Thrombocytopenia
    D. Polycythemia

67. Which one of the following oral conditions is not specifically characteristic of patients with HIV or AIDS?
    A. Herpes simplex
    B. Hairy leukoplakia
    C. Kaposi syndrome
    D. **Leukoedema**

68. Which term refers to a defect present at birth?
    A. Anomaly
    B. Inherited defect
    C. Congenital defect
    D. Developmental defect

69. A condition where two adjacent teeth are fused by only cementum is referred to as?
    A. Fusion
    B. Gemination
    C. Twinning
    D. **Concrescence**

70. A condition where a tooth with abnormal angulation or curve in the root or crown of a tooth is referred to as?
    A. Fusion
    B. Gemination
    C. Concrescence
    D. Dilaceration

71. Which of the following exhibit enlarged pulp chambers and short roots?
    A. Dens in dente
    B. Dens evaginatus
    C. Taurodontism
    D. Dilaceration

72. Which developmental anomaly is often associated with nonvital tooth and periapical lesions?
    A. Dens in dente
    B. Dens evaginatus
    C. Taurodontism
    D. Talon cusp

73. A tooth that is fused with the surrounding alveolar bone subsequent to the loss of intervening periodontal ligament is said to be
    A. Ankylosed
    B. Embedded
    C. Impacted
    D. Fused

74. Which of the following is not an odontogenic cyst?
    A. Dentigerous cyst
    B. Primordial cyst
    C. Median palatal cyst
    D. Lateral periodontal cyst

75. Enamel hypoplasia of a permanent tooth that results from infection of a deciduous tooth?
    A. Hutchinson's incisors
    B. Talon's tooth
    C. Turner's tooth
    D. Gorlin's tooth

76. A pear-shaped radiolucency causing displacement of roots of vital maxillary lateral and cuspid teeth is characteristic of:
    A. Globulomaxillary cyst
    B. Apical periodontal cyst
    C. Primordial cyst
    D. Nasoalveolar cyst

77. Features of multiple neurofibromas with cafe-au-lait spots of the skin are typical of:
    A. Von Recklinghausen's disease of skin
    B. Paget's disease of skin
    C. Hereditary ectodermal dysplasia
    D. Papillon-Lefevre syndrome

78. A cyst in the floor of mouth, caused by blockage of the salivary gland duct is:
    A. Follicular cyst
    B. **Ranula**
    C. Dermoid cyst
    D. Epidermoid cyst

79. All of the following developmental cysts of the jaw present as radiolucent lesions *except*
    A. Median palatal cyst
    B. Nasopalatine duct cyst
    C. **Nasoalveolar cyst**
    D. Globulomaxillary cyst

80. If a patient reports with excessive formation of scar tissue, it is called as:
    A. Myxoma
    B. Melanoma
    C. Carcinoma
    D. Keloid

81. A patient reported to dental clinic with white lesion on labial mucosa, cytological smear was taken. All of the following could be the diagnosis *except*
    A. Oral cancer
    B. Herpes zoster
    C. Lipoma
    D. Candidiasis

82. White, interlacing lines (Striae of Wickham) on the buccal mucosa and histologically civatte bodies, Max-Joseph space and saw-tooth rete ridges are characteristic features of:
    A. Leukoplakia
    B. Psoriasis
    C. Lichen Planus
    D. Carcinoma-in-situ

83. A patient reported to dental hospital with a painful growth associated with ulceration and itching of palate. On clinical examination, the paticnt had poor oral hygiene associated with two winged flies. What is the diagnosis?
    A. Actinomycosis
    B. Blastomycosis
    C. Cysticercosis
    D. Oral Myiasis

84. After an accident, a 4-year-old child visits to a dental hospital. On clinical examination you found the primary tooth intruded in to permanent follicle. It may result in
    A. Dens evaginatus
    B. Dens in dente
    C. Ankylosis
    D. Turner's hypoplasia

85. A 39-year-old black male reported to a dental hospital with slowly growing and bony expansion lesion in molar ramus area. On radiographic examination a multilocular cyst was noted & pathology report showed very coarse, granular, eosinophilic appearance of stellate reticulum cells which represented lysosomal aggregates. What could be the diagnosis?
    A. Ameloblastoma
    B. Dentigerous cyst
    C. Odontoameloblastoma
    D. Residual cyst

86. Which of the following organisms is responsible for progression of initial carious lesion into an extensive cavitation?
    A. Staphylococcus
    B. Streptococcus mutans
    C. Lactobacilli
    D. Streptococcus salivarius

87. Histologically majority of intraoral squamous cell carcinoma are:
    A. Carcinoma-in-situ
    B. Spindle cell type
    C. Poorly differentiated
    D. Well moderately differentiated

88. Few days ago a child patient reported with swelling in buccal and palatal maxillary anterior area. The radiograph showed a multilocular radiolucency. The pathology report suggested of giant cell in the lesion. What is the diagnosis?
    A. Giant cell fibroma
    B. Central Giant cell granuloma
    C. Hemangioma
    D. Peripheral giant cell granuloma

89. The risk for malignant transformation is greater in:
    - A. Speckled leukoplakia
    - B. Chronic hyperplastic candidiasis
    - **C. Erythroplakia**
    - D. Homogenous lichen planus

90. Person working in a pesticide chemical factory is more likely to get diagnosed histologically by which type of cell:
    - A. Tzanck cell
    - B. Ghost cell.
    - C. Neutrophil
    - **D. B cell & T cell lymphocytes**

91. A patient with slow growing, verrucous or warty patch with local destruction on tongue without any metastasis is likely to get confused histologically to:
    - A. Squamous cell carcinoma
    - **B. Benign epithelial hyperplasia**
    - C.
    - D. Spindle cell carcinoma
    - E. Melanoma

92. A 50-year-old female reported with a slow growing surface ulceration affecting accessory glands of palate which had recurred after surgical removal of the lesion. The pathology of the lesion showed basaloid epithelial cell nests that form multiple cyst like patterns that resembles a Swiss cheese pattern. The most likely diagnosis could be:
    - A. Pleomorphic adenoma
    - B. Mucoepidermoid carcinoma
    - **C. Cylindroma**
    - D. Acinic cell adenocarcinoma

93. A newly born child reports to a dental hospital with pedunculated lesion on crest of the maxillary alveolar ridge. The pathology report of the lesion showed sheets of large, closely packed cells showing fine, granular, eosinophilic cytoplasm with numerous capillaries. What could be the diagnosis?
    - A. Granular cell myoblastoma
    - **B. Congenital epulis of newborn**
    - C. Gingival cyst of newborn
    - D. Gingival cyst of adult

94. If a patient is suffering from slurring of speech, what is the diagnosis?
    - A. Strawberry tongue
    - B. Black hairy tongue
    - **C. Ankyloglossia**
    - D. Median rhomboid glossitis

95. A patient reported with a history of sensitivity and repeated exposure of teeth to vomiting. Identify what may be the result of this condition?
    - A. Abrasion
    - B. Attrition
    - **C. Erosion**
    - D. Caries

96. A 20-year-old boy underwent a restoration for decayed teeth. After few days he went for deep sea diving, where he experienced a toothache. This condition is referred as:
    - A. Chronic reversible pulpitis
    - B. Acute reversible pulpitis
    - **C. Aerodontalgia**
    - D. Focal reversible pulpitis

97. A 19 year old male patient presented with a swelling on the right side of the face. On clinical examination, 48 were unerupted and on radiographic examination, a pericoronal radiolucency was noticed. Histopathological examination showed that the epithelial lining was of variable thickness with certain few features resembling Gorlin and Vicker's criteria. The probable diagnosis is:
    A. Dentigerous cyst
    B. Adenaomatoid odontogenic cyst
    C. Unicystic ameloblastoma
    D. Ameloblastoma

98. A 25-year-old patient visited a dental clinic with an asymptomatic swelling in the lower left back tooth region. On a radiograph the third molar was impacted and associated with a radiolucent lesion. The most likely diagnosis considering the location alone is:
    A. Adenomatoid odontogenic tumour
    B. Periapical cemental dysplasia
    C. Ameloblastoma
    D. Odontoma

99. A 60-year-old patient presented with a swelling of the mandible in the left posterior region. On clinical examination, expansion of jaw, numbness and mobility of teeth were noted. X ray examination revealed multiple punched-out radiolucency were seen suggesting a diagnosis of:
    A. Multiple Myeloma
    B. Cleidocranial dysplasia
    C. Gardner's syndrome
    D. Paget's disease

References

Eversole. *Clinical Outline of Oral Pathology Diagnosis & Treatment* 3rd Edition.

Mervyn Shear. *Cysts of the Oral and Maxillofacial Region* 4th Edition.

Neville Brad. *Oral & Maxillofacial Pathology* 3rd Edition.

Rajendran. *Shafer'sText Book of Oral Pathology* 6th Edition.

Regezi. *Oral Pathology Clinical Pathologic Correlations* 6th Edition.

S. K. Purkit. *Essentials of Oral Pathology* 2nd Edition.

Saap Phillip. *Contemporary Oral Maxillofcail Pathology* 2nd Edition

Soames. *Oral Pathology* 4th Edition.

About the Editors

Dr. Mohammad Khursheed Alam, PhD

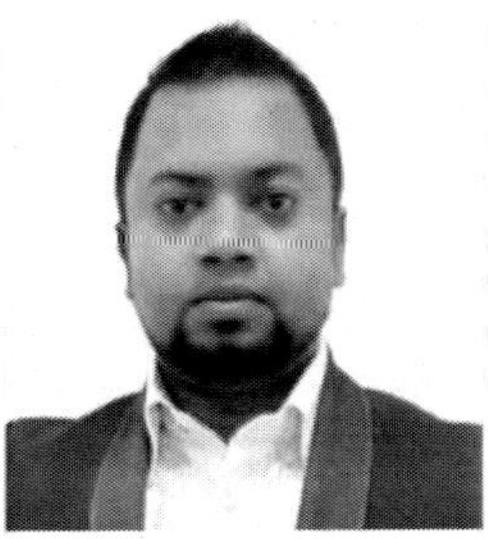

Dr. M. K. Alam is a Professor (Associate), Orthodontic Division, College of Dentistry, Jouf University (Since October 2016) and former Orthodontist at Orthodontic Unit, School of Dental Science, Universiti Sains Malaysia (5.6 years), HOD and Assistant Professor, at Department of Orthodontics, Bangladesh Dental College, Dhaka University (3.1 years). He received his dentistry training at University of Dhaka (2001) and his PhD in orthodontics from Hokkaido University, Japan (March 2008). His H index is 21 and RG score is 40.5 He has supervised more than 25 MSc, MOMSurg and PhD student as a main and co guide. Currently he is supervisor for more than 15 postgraduate students at school of dental sciences, Universiti Sains Malaysia with both national and international platform. He has both academic and clinical lead for orthodontics; with more than 600 publications and author for plenty of books and chapters. He is a member of the Editorial and Review Board of the many International and national Journal. He has been the invited speaker at several university orthodontic departments and guest speaker at lectures and courses worldwide.

Dr. Kiran Kumar Ganji, MDS

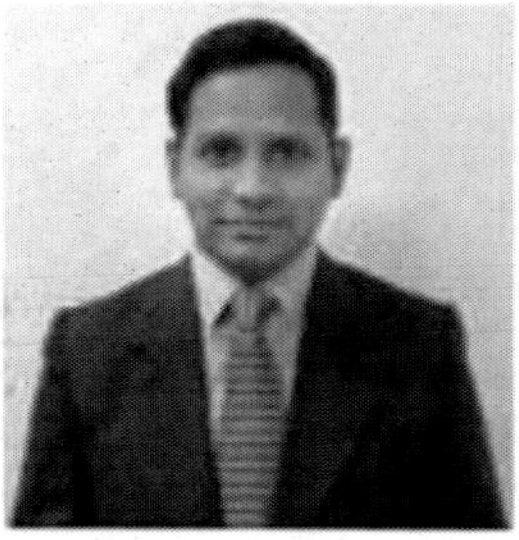

Dr. Kiran Kumar Ganji is an Assistant Professor and coordinator of Periodontics unit, College of Dentistry, Jouf University, Kingdom of Saudi Arabia. He received his dentistry training and his M.D.S in Periodontology & Implantology from Rajiv Ganji University of Health Sciences, Bangalore, Karnataka, India. His H index is 5 and RG score is 11.25. He is a member of the Editorial and Review Board of the many International and national Journal. He supervised for more than 10 postgraduate students at school of dental sciences with both national and international platforms. He has both academic and clinical lead for Periodontics he has more than 30 publications. His special interest is in periodontal regeneration and implant therapy.

Dr. Bader K. Alzarea MDSc, J. Board, GBOI

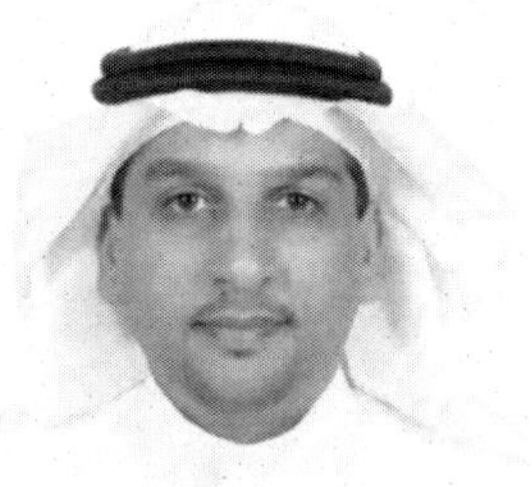

Dr. Bader K. Alzarea is the Dean of College of Dentistry and the Vice Rector of Jouf University, Sakaka, Kingdom of Saudi Arabia. He received his Master of Dental Science (MDSc) degree in Prosthetic Dentistry (Fixed & Removable) in 2004 from Jordan University of Science and Technology (JUST) and also cleared Jordanian Board in Prosthetic Dentistry (Fixed & Removable) in 2007and German Board of Oral Implantology (GBOI) in 2009. He obtained Implant Diploma from Toulouse University, France in June 2016. He got many publications in national and international journals having good impact factor. He is also an editorial and review board member of various renowned journals. He attended and presented posters at various national and internationally reputed conferences

Dr. Santosh R. Patil MDS

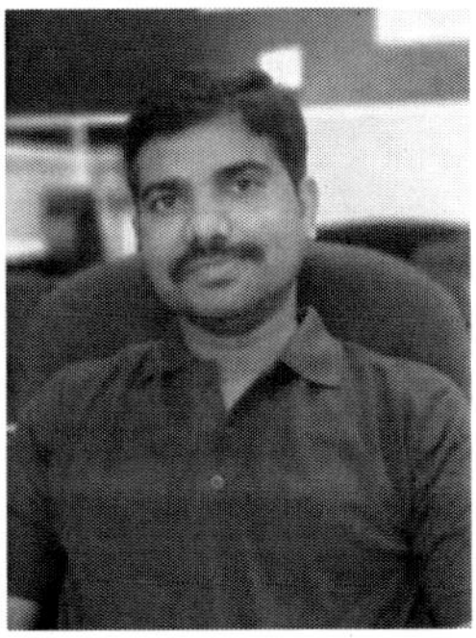

Dr. Santosh R. Patil completed his Masters in Oral Medicine and Radiology and currently working as Assistant professor and Head in Department of Maxillofacial surgery and diagnostic sciences, College of Dentistry, Jouf University, Kingdom of Saudi Arabia. He is a calibrated Oral Physician and maxillofacial radiologist with key interest in Oral Mucosal Lesions and 3D CBCT analysis of Craniofacial Structures including gender dimorphism and various soft and hard tissue pathologies. He has got numerous publications to his credit in various International and National Journals which are indexed in PUBMED, SCOPUS etc., and having Impact Factor. He authored textbooks which are very popular among the students.

Dr. Mohammed G. Sghaireen MDSc, J. Board, GBOI

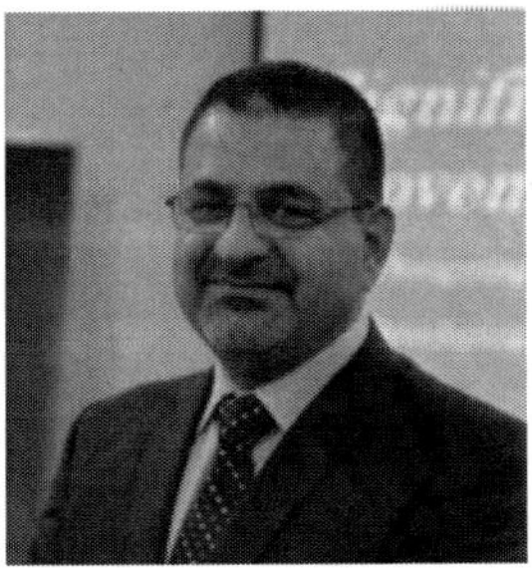

Dr. Mohammed G. Sghaireen is currently serving as Associate Professor and Head in Department of Prosthodontics. He completed his Master of Dental Science (MDSc) training in Prosthetic Dentistry (Fixed & Removable) in 2004 from Jordan University of Science and Technology (JUST) and cleared Jordanian Board in Prosthetic Dentistry (Fixed & Removable) in 2007and German Board of Oral Implantology (GBOI) in 2009. He completed Implant Diploma from Toulouse University, France 2016 and he is a fellow of International Academy for Dental-Facial Esthetics USA. He has published number of scientific articles in renowned journals.

INDEX

A

B

C

D

E

F

G

H

I

K

L

M

N

O

S

T

U

V

W

X

Z

Related Nova Publications

Dental Considerations for Medication-Related Osteonecrosis of the Jaw (MRONJ)

Author: Hani H. Mawardi

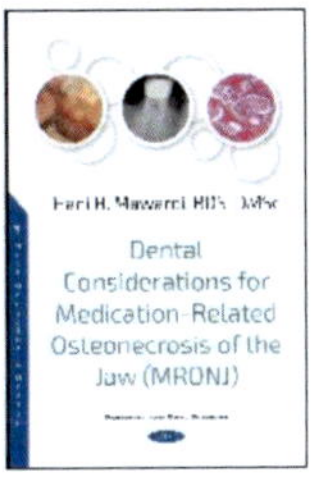

Series: Dentistry and Oral Sciences

Book Description: Dental Considerations for Medication-Related Osteonecrosis of the Jaw (MRONJ), First Edition provides a comprehensive review on MRONJ epidemiology, pathogenesis, clinical features, and diagnosis.

Softcover ISBN: 978-1-53613-755-2
Retail Price: $95

Bioactive Materials in Dentistry: Remineralization and Biomineralization

Editor: Francine Benetti, PhD

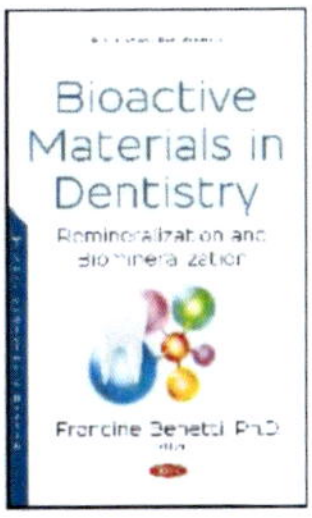

Series: Dentistry and Oral Sciences

Book Description: This book will address the use of different bioactive materials in dentistry, considering the performance of these biomaterials in the hard tissues of the tooth, and the response of the dental pulp, as well as the influence of the composition of these materials and of the individual's systemic alterations in bioactivity and in antimicrobial activity.

Hardcover ISBN: 978-1-53615-324-8
Retail Price: $160

Related Nova Publications

Periodontitis: Symptoms, Prevention and Treatment Options

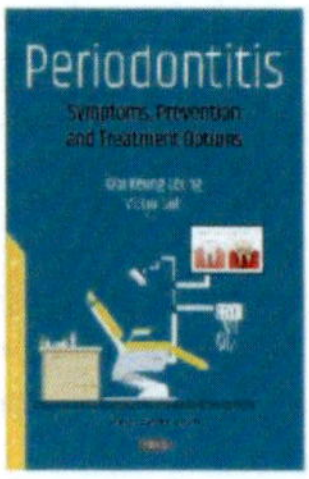

Authors: Wai Keung Leung and Victor Goh

Series: Dentistry and Oral Sciences

Book Description: Periodontitis is a bacteria initiated inflammatory disease of the tooth supporting structures. In the susceptible patient, progressive alveolar bone destruction often leads to tooth loss, exerting debilitating effects on one's overall quality of life.

Hardcover ISBN: 978-1-53615-154-1
Retail Price: $230

Case Reports in Dentistry

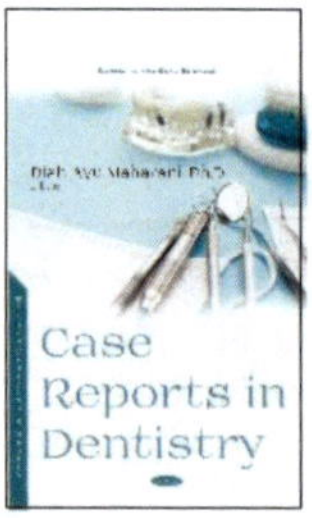

Editor: Diah Ayu Maharani

Series: Dentistry and Oral Sciences

Book Description: This collection of case reports in oral medicine, orthodontics, oral surgery, periodontology and prosthodontics addresses a number of clinical problems encountered in the treatment of various patients and shows how these cases have solved them.

Hardcover ISBN: 978-1-53613-303-5
Retail Price: $195